Healers & Heroes

ORDINARY PEOPLE IN EXTRAORDINARY TIMES

CLIF CLEAVELAND, MD, MACP

AUTHOR OF SACRED SPACE

AMERICAN COLLEGE OF PHYSICIANS
PHILADELPHIA

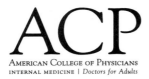

Manager, Books Program: Diane McCabe
Production Supervisor: Allan S. Kleinberg
Developmental Editor: Karen C. Nolan
Interior and Cover Design: Elizabeth Swartz
Composition: Wendy Smith

Printed in the United States of America by RR Donnelley

Library of Congress Cataloging-in-Publication Data
Cleaveland, Clif, 1936-   .
     Healers and heroes: ordinary people in extraordinary times / Clif Cleaveland.
         p. ; cm.
     ISBN 1-930513-54-2
     1. Medicine–Biography.   2. Medicine–Anecdotes.   I. Title.
     [DNLM: 1. Medicine–Biography. WZ 112 C623h 2004]
R134.C54 2004
610'.92'2–dc22

                                                            2004043716

04 05 06 07 08/10 9 8 7 6 5 4 3 2 1

For

Jane Plumlee, my nurse and dear friend for thirty-two years,

and

Marzena Lizurej and Barbara Kandora, my Polish friends,

who gave invaluable help to my study of Janusz Korczak

ACKNOWLEDGMENTS

I salute my teachers from first grade onward, who opened the magic of literature to me. The late Professor George Connor of the University of Tennessee at Chattanooga challenged me once to write a sustained narrative, and this led to my first book, *Sacred Space*. He encouraged my expansion of a series of lectures on medical heroes into this work. To me and many of my fellow physicians, George Connor and his UTC colleague, Gregory O'Dea, repeatedly emphasized the critical links between medicine and non-technical literature.

At the conclusion of each chapter I acknowledge the sources and persons from whom I derived information. The patience, helpfulness, and energy of these people — many of whom I had not met previously — were invaluable to my work.

Linda Smith, who manages my office, read and corrected my initial draft. Ruzha Cleaveland provided a meticulous review of the galley proofs, encouraged me onward when I hit barriers, and for forty-four years has made my life serene.

I am grateful to the books team at the American College of Physicians: my editor, Karen Nolan; Allan Kleinberg, who supervised production; Ed O'Rourke, for his marketing expertise; Elizabeth Swartz, who brought such pleasing design to the cover and the book's interior; Wendy Smith, compositor; and Diane McCabe, who presides over the books program. What a treat to work with them!

And I remain indebted to my heroes.

TABLE OF

CONTENTS

INTRODUCTION

ON THE BACKS OF HEROES

—∽∾∿—

I had a crush on Allene Hutchinson. She was my first grade teacher at Harwell Avenue School in LaGrange, Georgia. The photograph from my first day of school in September 1942 shows her, a prim brunette, standing next to me, her right hand resting on my right shoulder. She seems shorter in this picture than I remember. Tall for my age, as I would be for most of my years in grammar and junior high school, I stand to her right side, dapper in a necktie and a striped Palm Beach jacket. We did not have the word "blazer" in our 1942 vocabulary. Exposed wrists show that I am already outgrowing this coat. My legs appear scrawny below the hems of my short pants. My smile seems tentative. When I finished my assignments early, Mrs. Hutchinson gave me more columns to add and stories to read. She presided with gentle expertise over the launch of a twenty-two-year engagement with formal education.

After lunch each day, Mrs. Hutchinson read to us, usually one chapter per day, from books that usually required two or more weeks to complete. We were encouraged to rest our heads upon arms folded across the tops of our desks during the reading. Some of my classmates quickly fell asleep. I had difficulty containing my anticipation of the next installment in the current novel. *Lassie* left the most indelible imprint. This was the first long story that I had encountered that dealt with hardship and courage, the fortitude in this instance being demonstrated by a dog. I read and reread *Lassie* after receiving my own copy as a Christmas gift. I found comfort and inspiration in those first books.

Outside the classroom, I lived in fear. Gawky, nearsighted — a flaw that I concealed for years — and clumsy, I lived in fear of humiliation. When teams were picked or sides chosen for a playground game, I was the last person picked and sometimes was simply overlooked. I do not recall ever getting a hit when we played baseball. A beating at the hands of the older boys who presided over the hours outside the classroom constituted my biggest fear. During my elementary and junior high years, there were no social promotions. A student languished in a grade until he or she either met the requirements for promotion or attained age sixteen or married and left school. The first elopement of a classmate occurred in elementary school, she a mature, sweet-natured girl who wore faded sack-dresses.

I suspect that some of the older males at the Harwell Avenue School would be classified today as dyslectic or mentally impaired. They behaved in class under threat of being sent to the principal, a large and intimidating lady with the demeanor of a drill-sergeant. Legend had it that she wielded the paddle while the janitor held miscreants over a table. Recess was another matter. A number of retired, elderly teachers joined the faculty as replacements for younger teachers who relocated to be closer to their recently drafted husbands. A single teacher assumed playground duty each day. I doubt that some of the elderly monitors could see or hear very much of what transpired.

Like most of my peers, I sought anonymity within a group. Gangs of older boys terrorized any younger male whom they might isolate. A visit to the bathroom at recess was out of the question. We heard tales of frightening acts forced upon any younger boy who dared go to the toilet. Bladder control was essential.

Although threatened and chased from time to time, I was seriously accosted only once during my years in grade school, and that on a Halloween night. While trick-or-treating, two of us suddenly were surrounded by four of the dreaded older boys. They threatened to strip us, beat us, and lock us in the basement of a nearby church. One of our captors brandished a knife. My friend and I bolted to safety when a nearby porch light was turned on. A few days later I recognized one of the quartet when he came to our duplex to collect for our newspaper delivery. He told me that he would kill me if I ever revealed to my parents what had earlier transpired. I never saw him again. I assume he resigned his paper route.

Junior high school raised the level of risk. The older boys, now fully matured, became more blatantly threatening. We shared classrooms, locker rooms, hallways, and playgrounds with young men who routinely bragged of their sexual exploits and derided us mercilessly. Teachers avoided the backs of classrooms where sullen, older males slouched at their desks. Once, in a stairwell between classes, a classmate suffered a severe beating at the hands of a male several years his senior. His assailant attended class for two more days before the school board acted upon his expulsion.

I successfully maintained a low profile during school. I was not so fortunate during a weekend jamboree sponsored by the Boy Scouts. At the annual events troops competed against each other in a variety of outdoor contests such as map reading, first aid, and construction of rope bridges. I packed my camping gear — mess kit, sleeping bag, poncho, and other items purchased from an Army surplus store — and walked to the pickup point in the parking lot of my church. During the following day's competition in orienteering, my group came upon a fully operational liquor still. The nervous owner of the illicit distillery begged us not to report him. Of course, we did when we returned to our camp. Later, we were told that the proprietor and the most valuable parts of his equipment had disappeared by the time the sheriff acted upon our tip and raided the site.

After the day of competitions and a campfire, I walked toward the tent area. Suddenly, two older Scouts grabbed me, forced me to the ground, and shone a flashlight in my face. They blamed me for our troop's failure in one of the earlier contests of the day. I had no idea what they were talking about. I recall the beer on their breath. One of the pair held a knife against my throat while cursing me. An unknown voice firmly said, "Leave him alone," and my two assailants quickly withdrew. I never knew who intervened. I found excuses thereafter for not attending another scouting event. I kept my distance and avoided eye contact with my attackers. I had to maintain a higher level of vigilance. Fear left me a legacy of migraine.

My peers and I maintained a code of silence as far as telling our parents much of anything that occurred outside the classroom. Possibly, we thought that childhood and adolescence followed certain unchangeable patterns, and soon we would have completed our time of testing. In any event, we would with time acquire additional bulk and become more savvy in avoiding danger.

My protectors during those years were the real and fictional heroes whom I encountered in movies, books, and newspapers. World War II dominated the media during the first three years of school. I savored the exploits of aviators, tank crews, and submariners. An aunt gave me a history of a downed aircrew in the Pacific and their harrowing float to safety in a life raft. This was the first book of nonfiction that I read several times. I followed the course of the war in daily newspapers and broadcasts. I interpreted what I heard into piles of pencil drawings that invariably featured a hero engaged in battle with dastardly enemies. Intimidated at school, I could create a personal zone of safety in my imagination.

Heavily censored letters — V-mail — arrived from my mother's brothers who served overseas in the Army. Their reports and those passed through the family from cousins in North Africa, Italy, and France personalized the battles and presented me with heroes whom I knew. I searched an atlas to pinpoint their presumed duty stations.

Near the end of the war, my father received a letter from a friend of his who wrote from Iwo Jima. An infantryman, he wrote of his anticipation of returning to his civilian job. His letter arrived soon after my father learned that his friend had been killed in action. I assumed that this man whom I had met before his entry into military service had died heroically. This was the first fatality of war whom I had known.

My real and imagined heroes afforded me shelter in a childhood world that I found threatening and unpredictable. Each hero showed me an alternative to the fear in whose shadow I lived. I sensed that I might be able to borrow traits from my heroes so, if not heroic in my own right, I could at least conceal my doubts about my own worth.

Following junior high school, my family moved to Columbia, South Carolina, where danger seemed less prevalent. In this calmer venue, I continued to add to my personal hall of heroes. The Korean War supplied several. The televised Army-McCarthy hearings provided a civilian example of heroism in the person of Joseph Welch, who demonstrated to me the power of words in rebuffing an adversary, the Red-baiting Senator Joseph McCarthy. I learned that courage might take many forms beyond coping with physical dangers. I learned that heroic actions often occurred in quiet venues, with little or no acknowledgment and no thought of reward.

My heroes, in a way, delivered me safely through childhood and adolescence. They continue to guide and to inspire me. Subsequent years have revealed to me many instances in which people address and ultimately overcome obstacles of injustice, belligerence, ignorance, and illness.

I continue to build a complex mosaic of heroes. Several of their stories follow.

IN TIMES
OF WAR

Courage is rightly esteemed the first of human qualities . . . because it is the quality that guarantees the others.
— WINSTON CHURCHILL

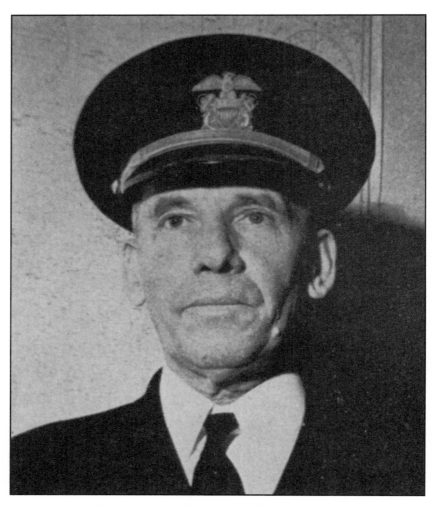

*Lieutenant Commander Corydon M. Wassell, MC, USNR, who received
the Navy Cross for his service to wounded crewmen from the
USS Marblehead and USS Houston.
(Photograph courtesy of Navy Medicine, Washington, D.C.)*

SEARCHING FOR
DOCTOR WASSELL

—◦⁄◦⁄◦—

War Movies

From the outset of World War II, movies drove our imaginations. Twelve cents purchased a seat for children aged twelve and under at the LaGrange Theater, and from 1942 onward our grammar school gang of nine missed few movies that dealt with the war. At least one new war movie opened each week.

Some of the earlier movies appeared in rose-tinted prints called sepia tone. With amateurish camera-work and little plot, the first harvest of war films casually rewrote history and delivered blatant propaganda, especially against the Japanese. Had a rating system existed, many of these movies would have earned an "R" or at least a "PG-13" designation for violent content. We sat enthralled, sometimes seeing the movie again the following afternoon before re-enacting the scenes in our wooded, kudzu-vined playgrounds. Our parents must have had other issues on their minds. I recall no enquiries about the movies we saw or their content. Birthday and Christmas presents of military paraphernalia abetted our movie-driven play. Wood and cardboard replicas of machine-guns, helmets, revolvers, and hand-grenades became our gifts of choice, our props for restaging the war. We assembled balsa models of Sherman tanks, B-25 bombers, and PT boats to use in tabletop war games. Pundits who speak of the benign influence of movies and television upon young minds are dead wrong.

On screen, atrocities were routine. Cowardly Japanese troops mutilated and blinded our soldiers, all of whom exhibited fortitude and patriotism. In one early film, a lone American pilot crashed his airplane into the funnel of a Japanese carrier. In another, an American, furious that his airbase had been strafed, gunned down the pilot of a Zero as he sought to escape his burning fighter. We not only pardoned but cheered the occasional atrocity committed by our side against a dastardly enemy. These early war films predominantly dealt with events in the Pacific. The movies were xenophobic to an extreme, reflecting the hatred directed in western states toward Japanese Americans. We absorbed and portrayed these attitudes in our re-enactments.

We watched as Robert Preston single-handedly held at bay Japanese invaders as they swarmed ashore on *Wake Island*. A patriotic message scrolled over the concluding battle implied that the Americans would fight to the last man. *Mrs. Miniver* portrayed the terrible impact of the London blitz upon civilians, including children, people who looked like us. At the end of that movie, Elgar's *Pomp and Circumstance* played while fighters of the Royal Air Force passed overhead, visible through the rafters of the bombed parish church. I think of this scene each time I hear *Pomp and Circumstance* at a high school or college commencement.

Wherever the theater of action, the American combat units featured similar compositions of slow-talking Southerners, wise-cracking New Yorkers, mid-Western farm boys with one resolute leader — John Wayne, Errol Flynn, or Humphrey Bogart — often misunderstood by his subordinates. Eventually the wisdom of the leader prevailed and evil was vanquished. The American military units contained no Latino or black personnel.

One movie of 1944 captured my attention like no other. Posters and previews billed *The Story of Doctor Wassell,* directed by the legendary Cecil B. DeMille, as a true account of a Navy surgeon charged with the care of badly wounded sailors in Java. Wassell, as portrayed by Gary Cooper, seemed tentative and vulnerable but utterly devoted to the care of his patients. Neither Japanese assault nor bureaucratic barrier could deter Wassell from the care of his men. The doctor had all the attributes of a saint, gently guiding others to safety despite hazardous circumstances and enormous obstacles. I watched the movie twice, but I do not recall ever re-enacting the plot. Perhaps it seemed sacred in contrast to the more typical shoot-'em-ups. After seeing the movie, I read in the *Atlanta Journal* of the real Dr. Wassell's popularity as he toured the country to promote the purchase of war bonds, and I added him to my personal panoply of heroes. The cinematic healer must have helped shape my vague yet evolving desire to become a physician.

Years later, while searching for a late-evening diversion on television, I encountered *The Story of Doctor Wassell* quite by chance on a classic movie channel. Though some of the scenes strained too hard to render patriotic images or comic relief — a Javanese nurse strips to a sarong to dance for the wounded sailors — the essence of heroic deeds by a noble physician remained. The doctor seemed fully believable.

The movie opens with an attack on an American cruiser, whose subsequently wounded soldiers travel by train to a hospital in the jungle of Java, where Dr. Wassell arrives to direct their care. When the Japanese invade Java, Wassell devotes himself to securing the safe passage of his patients to the coast for evacuation to Australia. Although some of the sailors are deemed too ill to transport, Wassell refuses to abandon them, remaining by their side until he is able to purchase deck space for them on a civilian steamer. War scenes alternate with flashbacks to pre-war China, where Wassell had served as a missionary before the war. The movie concludes with the awarding of the Navy Cross to Dr. Wassell.

Doctor Wassell: Childhood Hero

Post–World War II movies, freed of the need to stoke patriotism and hatred of our enemies, were free to explore the ambiguities and senseless acts and cruelties of warfare. In these renditions our heroes might be projected as deeply flawed individuals who were capable of cruelty as well as beneficence, cowardice as well as heroism. In light of such revisionist filmmaking, I wondered how closely *The Story of Doctor Wassell* approached the truth. I had to know if this icon of childhood would endure close scrutiny.

I recalled a book, *The Story of Doctor Wassell,* that I had read and reread at the time I had first seen the movie. Although my copy had been lost in various moves, a used book service located a copy for me.

Written by James Hilton in the spring of 1943, the biography spoke of Wassell in reverential tones. Lengthy interviews with the hero himself formed the basis of much of the narrative. Several of the wounded sailors were quoted as well. Book and movie were in reasonable accord, and I wondered if from its inception the book had been planned as a movie tie-in. As described by Hilton, Wassell seemed saintly and unencumbered by doubt. The sailors all came across as a band of wise-cracking adventurers.

I found a single reference to Dr. Wassell in Samuel Eliot Morison's *History of US Naval Operation in World War II:* ". . . Lieutenant Corydon M. Wassell of the Navy Medical Corps did wonders in evacuating the wounded and able-bodied by submarine or small Dutch merchantman." Although this is hardly the stuff upon which to build a movie, much less a legend, Admiral Morison's history did give me maps and descriptions of the naval actions in which Dr. Wassell figured. With the generous help of the Navy Medical Department, the library at the University of Arkansas, and surviving crewmen of the *USS Marblehead,* I embarked upon a study of my childhood hero.

Doctor Wassell: The Early Years

Corydon McAlmont Wassell was born on Independence Day 1884 in Little Rock. He began his premedical studies at Johns Hopkins University, returning to his home state to receive his medical degree in 1909 from the University of Arkansas.

For unknown reasons, Wassell's name was always misspelled in the *Cardinal,* the yearbook of the University of Arkansas. In those years, a slogan or motto accompanied the name of each medical student. For his sophomore year in 1907 Wassell was described as "A most pleasant gentleman at the City Hospital, the nurses say." In 1908 he was extolled as, "Star of his class, pride of the hospital." The class history and prophecy for "The Naught-Nine Cardinal" carried these comments:

> The historian writing the history of his class has a grievous and very much to be commiserated task, for it falls to his lot to be the sad recorder of the many who began and the few who finish, nor can he recall the blissful past without a melancholy sigh that it is gone forever . . . .

The fall of 1905 found this class composed of fifty-six members. Each succeeding year has been a winnowing of the wheat from the chaff. But twenty-four of the original fifty-six remain to-day. It has been a survival of the fittest.

According to one of the Profs, two members of this class are destined to become famous. Along what avocation was not stated, but from an intimate knowledge of the class born of four years' association, your prophet is assured that the fame of the favored two will not be gained in the realm of medicine. Hence this prophecy.

There are two ways by which men become famous. One is by thinking a little and by saying a great deal, and the other is by not thinking at all, and by saying nothing. And in accordance with the first many a vaporing, superficial individual acquires the reputation of being a brilliant man; and in accordance with the second many a block-head — like the owl, the most stupid of birds — is held a man of wisdom by a discerning world. 1929 will find two men of this class famous . . . .

Yet another has left the fold. Wasson [sic] has forsaken medicine for politics, in which new field he has become Justice of the Peace and his wisdom and his virtue are as those of Wouter Van Twiller . . . . [Van Twiller served an appointed term as governor of the New Netherlands Colony from 1633 until his removal in 1637. The biographical entry at Virtuology.com characterizes him as 'inexperienced in the art of government, slow in speech, incompetent to decide important affairs, and obstinate in minor matters.']

After graduation Corydon Wassell married and moved with his bride to Tillar, Arkansas, where he opened a private practice that steadily grew. In 1913 the young couple responded to the challenge of a visiting Chinese physician to become missionaries to China. Except for a brief furlough to the States in 1919, Dr. Wassell spent twelve years in China working variously as clinician, teacher, consultant and lecturer in neurology, and clinical investigator in parasitology. After his first wife died, he married an American nurse serving in China.

When his overseas obligations were concluded, Wassell returned to Arkansas. There were few jobs available for physicians, so he worked for the public school system in Little Rock, initiating vaccination and tuberculosis-screening programs. In 1936 he accepted an assignment as malaria control officer in a Louisiana camp for the Civilian Conservation Corps. Having previously joined the Naval Reserve, Wassell volunteered for active duty later that year. This was probably the most secure job that was available. He was fifty-two years old.

Wassell began active service as a member of an administrative panel at Key West. After the attack on Pearl Harbor, he received orders to assume managerial duties at a naval base at Surabaya, which was on the northern coast of Java, then part of the Dutch East Indies. On February 8, 1942, new orders directed his immediate departure by airplane for the inland town of Djokjakarta. Here he would serve as an administrative liaison for wounded American sailors who had recently arrived at the Dutch hospital in that town.

The Sea Battle Off Bali

In early 1942, Allied forces — British, Dutch, Australian, and American — retreated across the Pacific. Defeat loomed in the Philippines, and heavily guarded Singapore would fall in mid-February. A powerful enemy force approached the islands of Java and Sumatra, a prelude to multiple amphibious landings.

On February 4, a Dutch, British, and American flotilla of eight destroyers and four cruisers, including the US heavy cruiser *Houston* and the light cruiser *Marblehead,* sailed to intercept a Japanese convoy in the waters north of Bali. Without air cover, the mission had little prospect for success. The ships broke formation upon the appearance of the first wave of Japanese bombers, which attacked from high altitude. Swerving and twisting, the ships avoided the first clusters of bombs. In the fourth wave of enemy bombers, the *Houston* sustained a direct hit on her main deck. Fifty sailors were killed, and many others suffered serious burns. A near-miss seemed to lift the *Marblehead* from the water, and the concussion buckled the plates of her starboard bow. Observers aboard other ships assumed the *Marblehead* had sunk in clouds of smoke, but her ordeal was just beginning.

Launched in 1924, the 9500-ton-displacement *Marblehead* could achieve up to thirty-five knots and was highly maneuverable. Despite her best evasive actions, however, the *Marblehead* on this day received two direct hits, one wiping out her sick bay, the other peeling back the deck of her stern and locking her rudder hard left. The ship could sail only in tight circles, and water gushed through the hole in her bow. Her crew fought desperately to contain fires and keep their ship afloat. The attack killed fifteen and wounded thirty-four. Most of the wounded sustained burns of varying severity. Diesel fuel coated the decks where wounded were tended. Because most of the medical supplies had been lost in the explosion in the sick bay, crewmen had to improvise care for their wounded shipmates. Lubricating oils were applied to burns, and bed sheets served as dressings.

Barely afloat, her speed reduced to twelve knots, her rudder jammed, the *Marblehead* needed two days to limp through the strait between the islands of Bali and Lombok before turning westward for Tjilatjap on the southern coast of Java. The map of her journey resembles a corkscrew. Mercifully, no Japanese aircraft located the *Marblehead* during her slow and solitary voyage to safety. The *Houston* had reached Tjilatjap one day earlier and occupied one of the two floating dry docks in the harbor.

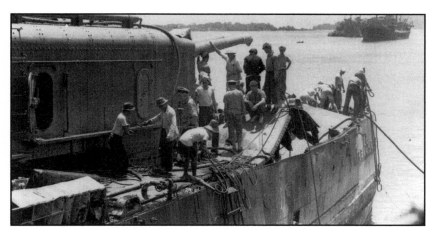

USS Marblehead at Tjilatjap, Java, after being damaged
by a Japanese air attack, February 4, 1942.
(Photograph courtesy of Department of the Navy, Washington, D.C.)

Still fearing attack by Japanese aircraft, the commanding officers of the *Houston* and *Marblehead* arranged for the transfer to shore of the most severely wounded sailors. The *Marblehead* lacked medical facilities and was barely seaworthy. The *Houston* anticipated an early return to battle and would need space for additional casualties. Repair crews worked frantically aboard both ships. Two days after the arrival of the *Marblehead*, both ships weighed anchor.

The *Houston* would be lost with most of her crew in the Battle of Sunda Strait off the northern coast of Java on March 1, 1942, joining a sad roster of Allied ships succumbing to superior Japanese weaponry. The *Marblehead* had been too badly damaged to be of further service. Her bow patched, she endured harrowing crossings first to Ceylon, then to South Africa, and finally across the Atlantic for definitive repairs. The *Marblehead* earned the nickname of "The Ship They Couldn't Sink." After extensive repairs, she served convoy duty for the duration of the war.

Tjilatjap had no American military hospital. Fifty-five wounded sailors, the majority of whom had come from the *Marblehead,* received dockside care before being placed aboard a hospital train for a journey of eight hours to a civilian hospital operated by the Dutch government in Djokjakarta. Here Dr. Wassell would meet his charges.

The Sailors Speak

With the assistance of Ray Kester, a veteran of the *Marblehead,* I located three sailors — Harold Holder, Oscar Rudie, and Walter Joyner — who had been under the care of Dr. Wassell in Java. I wrote each and requested an interview.

Harold Holder replied: "I don't feel I would be of any assistance to you. I was pretty much out of it during that period of time. About all I remember is people getting me out of Java, on a Dutch freighter, headed for Australia. From there it was back to the States and the Naval Hospital at Marc Island. Good luck in your endeavor."

Oscar Rudie in California agreed to a telephone interview. A twenty-year-old gunner's mate, he had been knocked unconscious by shrapnel that severely damaged an eye. Initially stretcher-bound, Rudie recalled the agonizingly long journey by train to the Dutch hospital, which was organized in a series of long, single-storied buildings, open at each end. Screens separated the sailors from native patients. Upon arrival, a Chinese surgeon, Dr. Yap, who was so diminutive that he stood upon a box to operate, tried to save Rudie's eye. These efforts failed, but Mr. Rudie recalled the skill and gentleness of the surgeon. As for Dr. Wassell, Mr. Rudie remembered a tall, slow-speaking officer, always in uniform, who wandered through the wards each day, visiting at the bedside of each American. Wassell smoked incessantly using a cigarette holder. He never seemed rushed.

I traveled to Baltimore to interview Walter Joyner. In a previous telephone call, he had urged me to hurry. "I have cancer, and I don't know how long I'll last." We met in the living room of his home. A trim, erect man with a fringe of silver hair, he had gathered photographs and military magazines for my review. He showed me a photograph of himself taken early in his naval career. The young man he had once been, in his starched, white uniform, bore a striking resemblance to the older veteran who now shared his story with me.

Joyner had enlisted in the Navy in 1940 at age eighteen. Aboard the *Marblehead* he served as a fireman in boiler room number two where he was responsible for lighting and maintaining three of the cruiser's twelve diesel-fired boilers. Top speed required the lighting of all twelve boilers. Firemen were sealed in below the waterline. They worked in intense heat. Upon the commencement of the enemy air attack, the bridge rang the engine room for full speed and power. Fireman Joyner felt the twists and turns of his ship as it took evasive action, and he felt the thuds of bombs falling far off target. Then a massive explosion occurred.

"Everything went black. I felt the whole ship had turned upside down. I don't know how the heck I got out of there. We were sealed in tight. Somebody had to carry me up ladders through narrow hatches."

Joyner had sustained wounds to his head and back. He lay upon a mattress on the deck, drifting in and out of consciousness during the two-day journey to Tjilatjap. Once aboard the hospital train he recalled being repeatedly kicked by the patient in the hammock beneath his. The journey seemed interminable. "The back of my head was all laid open, and I had shrapnel in my back."

An abiding memory of both Rudie and Joyner, however, was that of ice cream. A Christian evangelical group had visited the hospital one day, offering ice cream to any patient who would make a profession of faith. Walter Joyner remembered: "They tried to push religion down our throats, and some of the boys told them to go to hell. They left without giving us any ice cream."

When on the following day Wassell learned of the incident, he procured from a shop in the town ice cream for every patient in the hospital, sailor and native alike. The frozen treat cemented a tight relationship between the sailors and Dr. Wassell.

Joyner improved rapidly and could soon move about the hospital without assistance. Once sailors became ambulatory, they assisted in the care of those men confined to bed.

One day Dr. Wassell recruited Joyner to accompany him on a trip to the town's brewery where Lieutenant Commander Wassell treated Fireman Joyner to a beer. The two men brought several cases of beer to the hospital for their comrades.

Both Rudie and Joyner recalled the ingenuity of Dr. Wassell in addressing the smoking needs of the burned sailors. Because of bulky dressings on their hands and arms these men had to rely upon nursing staff to light and manipulate their cigarettes. Wassell commissioned the carving of extra-long cigarette holders that would extend beyond the foot of each patient's bed. Nurses could attach a cigarette, light it, and then go about their duties because the long holders precluded any risk that bedclothes might be accidentally set afire.

When air raid sirens sounded, ambulatory sailors carried those who remained bedfast from the ward into sandbagged bomb shelters. A team of four men transported each of the severely burned patients. Despite best efforts at gentleness, Joyner sensed that such movement caused great pain to these patients.

At night Joyner and other ambulatory patients helped the nurses, half of whom were Dutch, half Javanese, in washing, drying, and rolling dressings. "Those nurses, they were the real angels," recalled Joyner. He often wondered what became of the hospital's staff after the Japanese army overran the town.

Meanwhile, Japanese forces had landed on nearby Borneo and Sumatra. Java would be next. In mid-February, Wassell received orders to evacuate the ambulatory patients to Tjilatjap where they would board ships bound for Australia. Bedfast patients would be left behind.

Ignoring the directive, Wassell loaded *all* of his patients aboard the hospital train for the journey to the coast.

Chaos reigned in the port city. Joyner was assigned a berth on the oiler *USS Pecos.* A sailor who had been assigned space on the *USS Sturgeon,* a submarine, approached Joyner to trade places with him. The thought of passage on a submarine terrified the sailor, so Joyner agreed to switch places and departed Java aboard the *Sturgeon.* The submarine would detour to Corregidor to rescue several nurses from that besieged fortress. The vessel was so crowded that there was barely space to sit, but Joyner landed safely in Australia. After further convalescence and the issuance of new uniforms and papers, he resumed active duty at sea. He retired in 1960 after twenty years of active duty.

The *Pecos,* which had provided passage for many Allied evacuees, was sunk by an enemy torpedo soon after her departure from Java. Oscar Rudie, one of the fortunate walking-wounded, sailed for Australia aboard another vessel. Nine stretcher-bound patients, however, were turned away at dockside. Officers in charge argued that helpless patients would jeopardize the safety of other personnel in the likely event of a torpedo attack. Wassell chose to remain with these patients. Because the hospital train had departed, Wassell had to purchase space for his patients aboard a freight train for the return to Djokjakarta. The staff at the hospital welcomed the returning Americans. In the ensuing days, the town and hospital came under daily air attack, but none of the patients suffered injuries in these raids.

With the invasion of Java imminent, Dr. Wassell negotiated space for his patients in a British motor convoy bound for Tjilatjap. The British troops had been ordered to establish a defensive perimeter around the port. Wassell drove one of the trucks. To avoid air attack, the convoy took a circuitous route over narrow roads overhung with dense foliage. Repeatedly, enemy aircraft passed overhead, fortunately never spotting the trucks. Because of intolerable pain one sailor asked to be left at a wayside first-aid station. Wassell reluctantly agreed to leave him behind; the sailor later reached safety. Wassell and his eight patients reached Tjilatjap after two days on the road. The port had been heavily bombed during the previous night, and only two ships remained at anchor in the harbor.

Doctor Wassell contacted a Captain Prass, who commanded one of the ships, a Dutch inter-island passenger steamer, *M/S Janssens*. After protracted negotiations, Wassell purchased deck space for his men aboard the *Janssens,* which would sail the next morning. Six hundred passengers crammed into a space designed for one third that number. Tjilatjap would fall to Japanese invaders eight days later.

Seeking to avoid submarine and air attack, Captain Prass followed a roundabout route to Australia. Even so, *Janssens* came under repeated strafing attacks by Japanese Zeroes. Remarkably, only one passenger was wounded during these attacks. A near rebellion by a number of passengers resulted in their being put ashore on a small island. The *Janssens* sailed on and reached Freemantle after a voyage of slightly over two weeks.

Doctor Wassell's patients remembered his unceasing attention to their comfort and safety throughout the voyage. Of the entire contingent of wounded sailors who were transferred ashore from the *Houston* and *Marblehead,* only one succumbed to his injuries.

The President Addresses the Nation

On April 28, 1942 President Roosevelt addressed the nation by radio. After outlining the setbacks in the first five months of the war and the duties of those on the home front, the President presented two stories of valor:

> There is, for example, Dr. Corydon M. Wassell. He was a missionary, well known for his good works in China. He is a simple, modest, retiring man, nearly sixty years old. But he entered the service of his country and was commissioned a Lieutenant Commander in the Navy.

After summarizing the events at the Dutch hospital, Roosevelt described the overland evacuation to Tjilatjap:

> He had to get the twelve men to the seacoast — fifty miles away. To do this, he had to improvise stretchers for the hazardous journey. The men were suffering severely, but Dr. Wassell kept them alive by his skill, and inspired them by his own courage.

And as the official report said, Dr. Wassell was "almost like a Christ-like shepherd devoted to his flock."

Describing the evacuation by Dutch ship, Roosevelt concluded:

> A few days later, Dr. Wassell and his small band of wounded men reached Australia safely. And today Dr. Wassell wears the Navy Cross.

The Navy Cross is second only to the Medal of Honor as an award for valor in the Navy or Marine Corps. Corydon Wassell earned this decoration, despite disobeying orders, by ensuring the safe passage of all the patients entrusted to his care.

Doctor Wassell completed his military service in stateside assignments. These included numerous appearances at which he promoted the purchase of war bonds. Corydon Wassell retired from the Navy with the rank of Rear Admiral. He died in 1958 and is buried in Arlington National Cemetery.

★   ★   ★

In 1944 Walter Joyner visited Chicago during a two-week furlough. He invited a date to accompany him to a movie, *The Story of Doctor Wassell*. Almost sixty years later as I sat with him in his living room in suburban Baltimore, Mr. Joyner reported, "Doc, I had to get up and leave halfway through. It wasn't like that at all. It wasn't like that at all."

★   ★   ★

I did not know what I might find when I began my enquiry into the wartime deeds of Dr. Wassell. Movies, after all, are notorious for taking liberties with history and biography. *The Story of Dr. Wassell* captured the traits — optimism, dedication to his patients, and sensitivity to their needs — so respected by veterans Rudie and Joyner, but the movie played loosely with the facts in two evacuations of the wounded by truck and by boat.

Neither survivor recalled an occasion when Dr. Wassell performed surgery or changed dressings for the wounded sailors. Rather, through his deliberate and relaxed daily rounds in the hospital he sustained hope and addressed in other ways the physical and emotional comfort of his

15

charges. Oscar Rudie remembered Dr. Wassell "looking and talking and checking all the time." He assumed the role of father for his men.

The ice cream that Dr. Wassell procured for each of the hospital's patients forms the most enduring memory for the retired sailors. The long, custom-carved cigarette holders probably brought similar relief to the men who could not use their arms. Cold beer added another touch of the homes they longed to see. In none of the dealings with the wounded sailors did rank create a barrier. I can imagine Dr. Wassell saying, "We are all in this together, and we will all get out of this together."

My study uncovered many heroes. The commanders of the various Allied warships did not hesitate to sail into battle against desperate odds. Aboard the *Marblehead,* one or more anonymous rescuers pulled Walter Joyner from the darkened and damaged boiler room. While the fate of the *Marblehead* remained precarious, the needs of the wounded lying upon her decks were never overlooked. Nurses and physicians at the Dutch hospital did not waver in their provision of expert, loving care for these foreign sailors suddenly thrust into their facility. Against a backdrop of steadily worsening reports from the frontlines, the hospital team sustained without panic or despair their mission to heal the wounded and sick, whether native Javanese or American sailor. I have so far found no materials in English that record the fate of the hospital and its staff.

The wounded sailors never lost hope that they would reach safety. Ambulatory patients assisted in the care of their badly wounded comrades in the burn ward. Oscar Rudie requested transfer into that ward so that he could comfort a friend. "It wasn't so bad, once you got used to the smell," he recalled. The challenge of keeping up with the need for clean dressings could not have been met without the nightly efforts of those sailors less wounded. When air attacks threatened, the walking wounded ensured that no patient would be left in the wards; all would be carried to shelter no matter the risk to personal safety.

In a career characterized by repeated examples of selfless service, Dr. Wassell established an unforgettable standard for devotion to his patients. When orders arrived to move only ambulatory patients to the coast, he chose to evacuate all of his patients. So easily he could have carried out the orders to the letter, assuming that the bedfast patients would eventually find some transport to safety. At the dockside of the port city of Tjilatjap, he could have left the badly wounded sailors behind with an assurance that someone else would intervene on their behalf to find a means of escape, but Dr. Wassell refused to delegate responsibility for the safety of his patients. He was their physician, and he would personally see to their safe passage. He would not break the trust that his patients placed in him.

In my hometown an ice company advertised, "Weighed, found not wanting." I asked my parents what the slogan meant. They replied that the company guaranteed that their blocks of ice were accurately measured. In the manner of the long-defunct ice company, I affix to Dr. Wassell, my earliest hero, "Studied, found not wanting." In fact he turned out to be far more courageous than I could have anticipated.

SOURCES AND ACKNOWLEDGMENTS

The Story of Doctor Wassell (1943) by James Hilton was the basis of the 1944 movie (available on VHS tape). Cassandra McCraw, Reading Room Supervisor for the Special Collections Division of the University of Arkansas Libraries, supplied a photograph of Dr. Wassell, relevant text from the 1909 *Cardinal* (yearbook), and useful background information. Jan Herman, editor of *Navy Medicine,* provided a photograph of Dr. Wassell in uniform, copies of letters from Wassell to the Dutch Ambassador to the United States and to Queen Wilhelmina of the Netherlands, and a summary of Wassell's service record. For a detailed history of the naval battles around Java, I depended upon Samuel Eliot Morison's *History of United States Naval Operations in World War II, volume 3, The Rising Sun in the Pacific* (1948). Admiral Morison's fifteen-volume history is endlessly fascinating in its detailed and humane accounts of the war at sea. The Web site for the *USS Marblehead* led me to Ray Kester of the Marblehead Association. He in turn placed me in contact with veterans Harold Hunter, Oscar Rudie, and Walter Joyner, the last of whom gave me copies of a map of Djarkajota (which he carried with him when he was evacuated), a photograph of the *Marblehead,* and various articles related to the cruiser's travails. Further information and the photograph of the *Marblehead* used here came from the Web site of the Naval Historical Center, Department of the Navy, Washington, D.C.

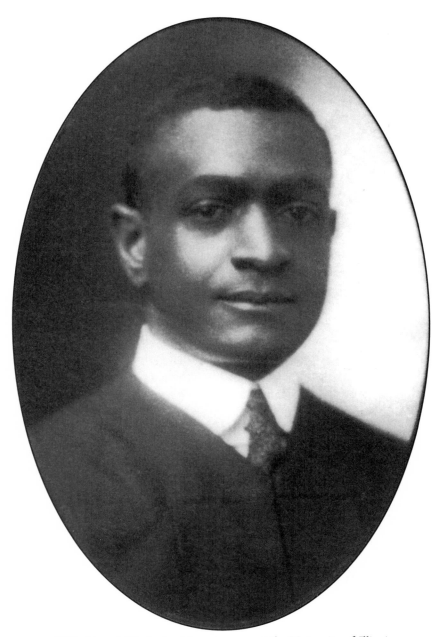

Billie Dyer, MD, during his senior year at the University of Illinois College of Medicine, 1916. (Photograph courtesy of Douglas Becknese, Curator, Richard J. Daley Library, University of Illinois at Chicago.)

THAT DEMOCRACY
MIGHT REIGN: THE STORY
OF BILLIE DYER

—◁◦◦▷—

I could not find the cemetery. Either the directions were faulty or my navigational sense had failed. Twice I had asked its whereabouts from people on the street, and twice I had received different instructions on how to get there. Finally, I found the old city cemetery of Lincoln, Illinois. A caretaker at the office looked up the name I had requested, *William Holmes Dyer*, and pointed out his gravesite on a large framed map. A short drive along the winding single-lane road, and I was there. After brushing dead leaves and dirt from the headstone, I stood awhile and thought about the man beneath this sod. I considered him a friend and an inspiration, although we had never met – in person.

I first was introduced to Dr. Dyer in a 1992 collection of short stories by William Maxwell, *Billie Dyer and Other Stories*. Maxwell had previously captured my admiration with *So Long, See You Tomorrow*, his 1979 novel that remains almost too painful to read in its description of friendship and its loss. The stories in the later volume were no less powerful. Memory and imagination blend seamlessly in the writings of Maxwell. As he writes in "Billie Dyer," "For things that are not known — at least not anymore— and that there is now no way of finding out about, one has to fall back on imagination. This is not the same thing as the truth, but neither is it necessarily a falsehood."

Maxwell's title story focuses on Billie Dyer, a black physician whose father was the grandson of slaves and whose mother was the daughter of slaves. Born in Lincoln, Illinois in 1886, William H. Dyer graduated from Lincoln High School. Several years passed before he was able to begin his three years of undergraduate study at Lincoln College. He earned his medical degree at the University of Illinois at Chicago in 1916. His senior year photograph shows a serious demeanor with a powerful gaze. Billie Dyer was in his thirtieth year as he began his internship in Kansas City. After this year of postgraduate training, he opened a general practice in his hometown, but with America's entry into the First World War, he volunteered for Army service.

Doctor Dyer kept a diary during his eighteen months of service in the Medical Corps. Years after his death in 1958, the diary found its way to the Public Library in Lincoln. A browser at a flea market in Texas had purchased the handwritten journal and, thinking that it might be of interest to the citizens of Lincoln, forwarded the diary to the library. Through the kindness of Richard Sumrall, Director of the Lincoln Public Library, I obtained a copy. I was struck by the legibility of the handwriting, so unlike the scrawl that so many of us call script today. William Maxwell had quoted accurately from the diary's hundred pages and had selected many poignant passages for his narrative. The diary plus Dyer's attached military record portrayed a man of dignity and quiet courage. I needed to learn more.

In preparation for my visit to Lincoln, I contacted Dr. Dyer's undergraduate alma mater and met Debbie Ackerman, the director of Lincoln College's Office of Advancement. Her office was the first stop during my day-long visit to Lincoln. She and her staff surprised me with a copy of Billie Dyer's academic transcript. During his three years of study, from 1910 to 1912, Billie took courses in Latin, German, and science. His numeric grades ranged from a seventy-five in German to a ninety-one in science. Because he would have been twenty-four when he entered Lincoln College, I presumed that Billie had had to work for several years to afford collegiate study.

Lincoln, Illinois has the distinction of being the first American city named for our sixteenth President before his inauguration. Founded in 1853, the town lists William Maxwell and Langston Hughes among its sons. I located the house in which William Maxwell had lived, but I could not determine where Billie Dyer had resided.

Unfortunately, my plans to examine the original diary fell through because the library was closed on the Friday of my visit. Although I decided that that treat would have to await my next trip to Lincoln, at least I had a copy of the diary, a novella based upon that diary, an undergraduate transcript, a graduation photograph from medical school, and a gravesite for the biography I wished to write. I was reminded of connect-the-dots puzzles for children, only my present challenge was without all of the dots.

Despite the fact that black Americans had fought in the Revolutionary War and the Civil War, their status remained tenuous in the American army. Upon entry into World War I in 1917, the United States required registration of all able-bodied men aged twenty-one to thirty-one, and, although some recruiting stations denied African Americans the opportunity to join the Army, eventually seven hundred thousand registered. Almost three hundred seventy thousand African Americans entered active duty. The great majority of these soldiers served in supply, labor, and service jobs. Fatal clashes occurred at multiple sites in the South between white and black soldiers and between black soldiers and white civilians. The Army created two new all-black combat divisions. The 92nd Division served under the US flag and was composed of draftees. The 93rd Division consisted primarily of National Guard units and served under French command. Dyer, commissioned a First Lieutenant upon enlistment, was assigned to the 317th Ammunition Train of the 92nd Division.

He wrote of his enlistment: "I had just completed my internship at the Kansas City General Hospital and returned home to begin my practice of medicine. Each day the call became more urgent for young men between the ages of twenty-one and thirty-one years to defend the colors and with thousands of others, I decided to offer my life upon our Nation's altar as a sacrifice, that Democracy might reign and autocracy be forever crushed." Throughout the diary Dr. Dyer uses the term "colored" when writing about members of his race.

On July 26, 1917, Dyer received notification from the Surgeon General of the Army that he met the qualifications for active duty.

A subsequent letter from the Department of the Army documented his appointment as a First Lieutenant in the Medical Reserve Corps. Hundreds of friends and fellow citizens of Lincoln, Illinois gathered at the train depot on September 24 to bid their farewell to the young physician as he departed for Fort Des Moines, Iowa. Tears continued to spill from Dr. Dyer's eyes long after his train had pulled away from the station.

Dyer joined a company of 300 black officers at Fort Des Moines. This was one of several military posts in the North and Midwest where components of the 92nd Division would train. Not until the concluding weeks of the war would all elements of the division serve in a unified command. Dyer endured the first of several affronts upon his arrival at Fort Des Moines: his quarters consisted of an unheated room in a stable. Then and subsequently he focused on a larger challenge. "I was in the Army to do my bit to make the world safe for Democracy."

His days consisted of four hours of drill followed by four hours in the classroom to learn "that most difficult of all branches, the Army paper work." Repeated drill suggests that the Army had no clear idea as to how the black medical officers would be utilized.

Many of Dr. Dyer's fellow officers received orders assigning them to other bases; he and twenty comrades remained behind. Drill and classes continued. On November 12, the group received orders to travel at once to Camp Funston, Kansas where he and his fellow officers again joined a unit of the 92nd Division. Pausing in Kansas City, Dr. Dyer re-established contact with Bessie Bradley, a teacher whom he had met during his year of internship. They would secretly marry in Alton, Illinois on March 6, 1918.

Drill and lectures continued; this time around, enlisted men participated in the classes. On December 1 headquarters assigned Dr. Dyer to the infirmary of the 317th Ammunition Train. This unit would provide both shells for artillery and ammunition for small arms borne by infantrymen. Finally, Dyer could cease the repetitive lectures and drills and work as a physician. Examinations of incoming recruits occupied his days until an epidemic of meningitis erupted in January. The medical officers worked day and night to cope with a flood of very ill patients. No antibiotics existed at that time. Contemporary therapies included potassium bromide for relief of headaches and repeated lumbar punctures to relieve excessive pressure of cerebrospinal fluid. The only other therapy in wide use at the time consisted of prolonged soaks in hot baths, a treatment advocated by Sir William Osler, the most distinguished physician in the English-speaking world. Many soldiers died in the barracks in which they were quarantined. Survivors often remained so weak that they could not resume active duty for many weeks. Healthy soldiers received daily nasal sprays of disinfectant solutions. The frightful epidemic finally subsided after several harrowing weeks.

On June 6, orders arrived for the movement of the medical unit to Camp Upton on Long Island to prepare for embarkation to Europe. Dyer and his comrades sailed on the *Covington,* one of several troopships accompanied across the Atlantic by two battleships and several destroyers. On board were five thousand troops, including the all-black 366th infantry regiment and the all-white 115th National Guard Unit.

"Soon we passed that most honored, most noble of monuments, the Statue of Liberty." Liberty, however, did not extend to the ship's company. "From the very start there was that feeling of prejudice brought up between the White and Colored Officers, for among the first orders issued were those barring Colored Officers from the same toilets as the Whites, also barring them from the barbershop and denying Colored Officers the use of the ship's gymnasium."

The days at sea consisted of segregated sick call and endless sanitary inspections. After the *Covington* docked at Brest on June 27, Dyer and his unit marched several miles inland to the Pontenaizen Barracks, "a terrible and dirty old place," used in the time of Napoleon as a prison. Dyer uncovered within the buildings a variety of instruments that had been used in the torture and execution of prisoners. At each stop, he acquired bits of local lore. En route to the Pontenaizen Barracks he noted an abiding sense of mourning among a civilian population composed almost entirely of women and children.

At each posting in France, Dr. Dyer studied the history and architecture of his surroundings. "During my stay in Brest, I succeeded in getting passes to the City on two afternoons for I was extremely anxious to see more of the strange old City. The people, direct descendents of the Britons, have all strange and antique customs . . . I spent a couple of hours in a park one afternoon and almost immediately when I was seated upon a bench the young children began to congregate around me not even attempting to be one bit timid. Soon they were sitting upon my knees and pointing to my eyes, nose and ears trying to teach me the French words for the same."

On July 4, Dr. Dyer and his fellow soldiers entrained to Montmorillon. The train stopped miles short of its destination, and the soldiers were ordered to leave their coaches at once. A long march followed. At Montmorillon, Dyer and the other officers were assigned quarters in estate homes whose owners were away. The enlisted men lived in tents. Days for the doctor consisted of more drill and sick-call in the infirmary. Evenings brought the officers into contact with the residents of the town.

"In the large library was an old piano and often in the evening the peasant French women living in the adjoining estate would come over and sing for us and try to teach us their latest country dances. At St. Laomir, a small village nearby, we met the family of the schoolmaster at whose home we were pleasantly entertained. We being the first American troops in this area, the people soon fell in love with us . . . . We found these people to be extremely fine and what pleased us most, there was no thought of prejudice for with them there was No Color Line." At no point in the diary did he note attitudes of racism among French citizens.

Fresh orders on July 22 assigned Dr. Dyer to two companies that would travel by train to Marseilles to pick up ammunition trucks that they would drive northward to rejoin their parent unit. Officers traveled in coaches. Enlisted men were jammed into freight cars. Dyer observed no young men and no horses en route. He presumed that all had been sent to the front lines.

After his arrival at the Mediterranean coast four days later, Billie wrote, "The population of Marseilles seems to be one great conglomeration of races. It seems that God just transplanted a sample of his people from all kingdoms of the earth in this strange old city." Algerians in red skull-caps mingled with turbaned Hindus in loose garments.

"The French people here as in every other part of the county were extremely friendly and regarded us curiously, we being the first colored American officers they had ever seen . . . . We found a welcome in the best hotels, cafes, theaters, in fact everywhere, for the French have no prejudice."

In Marseilles, and whenever possible at the multiple stops of his European tour, Dr. Dyer delighted in visits to public gardens and historic shrines. He collected postcards and other pictures of each city and attached these to the pages of his diary. He analyzed the people and their customs. In Marseilles he observed widespread and quite public prostitution and excessive drinking in and around multiple saloons. The permanent residents of Marseilles consisted only of women, children, and old men. Whenever he saw young Frenchmen, they were in uniform, moving in slow processions toward the stale-mated combat zones.

No trucks could be found for transporting ammunition, so the unit planned its return. The detachment entrained first for Dijon before joining on August 5 the same elements of the 92nd Division that Dyer had first encountered at Camp Des Moines and Camp Funston. The Army clearly had not yet devised a definite mission for this division whose units continued to arrive in France until October. A week later the unit finally received orders to proceed by truck to Bruyeres, near the front lines. Perhaps a mission of some consequence awaited the soldiers.

"Buckling my pistol to my side I started on my mad hunt for the Germans." At night Dyer felt the concussions and watched the flashes from a bombardment of nearby Epinol by German aircraft. "Apart from some humiliating divisional orders our stay was most pleasant." The source of the humiliation remains unclear.

The 92nd Division moved by truck to Raon L'Etape in the Vosges Mountains of northeastern France, traveling though a devastated country-side of abandoned trenches, shell craters, and destroyed villages and farm-houses. French and American infantrymen trudged past. The black soldiers bivouacked in the woods, aware each day of German aircraft cir-cling overhead. Dyer and the other medical officers moved into the home of a French woman for a month. He attended a burial ceremony for two German fliers who had been killed in the crash of their bomber. An honor guard of French and African American soldiers accompanied the caskets. Once the coffins had been lowered into their graves, a French priest offered prayers. "As I stood and watched it all — how cold, how sad, I could not but have a feeling of sympathy for they were some Mother's boys."

In the Vosges sector, the 317th Ammunition Train saw its first real action, supplying artillery shells for the 92nd Division and for French batteries. Because of the risk of air attack, the transfer of ammunition had to be carried out at night. The 317th next marched into the Argonne Forest where the troops worked continuously, providing ammunition for infantry regiments of the 92nd Division. Soon after this action, Dr. Dyer read with disbelief a bulletin from division headquarters: "Negro soldiers will be used to handle the mustard-gas cases because the Negro is less susceptible than the Whites."

The 317th next moved into dilapidated French barracks at St. Mine-feld, site of a graveyard for six thousand French soldiers. On October 7, the various components of the 92nd Division congregated at Belleville where infantry and artillery companies that had been training in Southern France joined the force. The journey to Belleville took Dr. Dyer through a landscape of complete devastation. Hardly a tree remained standing. At night the motor convoy inched forward in snow and fog. Finally, in Belleville, the division reached full force. Its exact mission remained elusive. Belleville was within artillery range of Metz, still held by German forces. The dreaded enemy bombardment never found its mark, although enemy artillery rounds whistled overhead during most nights before exploding just beyond the town's perimeter. Dyer set up his dispensary in an abandoned electrical plant where he worked at an exhausting pace to treat the respiratory illnesses that afflicted troops bivouacked in constant cold and rainy weather. Rumors of peace alternated with rumors of a final assault upon German fortifications at Metz.

On November 8, Dyer wrote, "While we were in the midst of our activities a terrible thing occurred at Belleville which dampened our ambitions. A colored boy who had been convicted of rape in August was hanged or lynched in an open field not far from my infirmary. The execution was a military order but so openly and poorly carried out that it was rightly termed a lynching."

The following day, the 92nd Division responded to orders that directed a full-scale attack upon Metz. "Tremendous barrages were laid down by our Artillery in support of our infantry's advances." In fighting its way into the outskirts of Metz, the 92nd Division sustained heavy casualties in what would be the final battle of World War I. News of the signing of a peace accord reached the 92nd Division on November 11. Fighting abruptly ceased. "Bells rang, whistles blew, men, women and children shouted for joy at the ending of the World's greatest conflict and the winning of the Right."

Dyer returned to Belleville where he shared with another lieutenant a second floor room in an ancient, dilapidated house. "Above us was a loft full of straw in which many rats, mice and birds were quartered, they often put on jollifications and threw chaff upon us quite to our disgust."

On a brief furlough on December 6, Dr. Dyer and a friend toured the ruined landscape around Metz. Fresh graves alongside the road reminded Dyer of the cost of victory. "Fields bitterly covered with shell holes, trenches, machine gun nests, barbed wire entanglements for a solid stretch of fifteen miles. This whole region was a barren waste and showed all evidences of modern warfare. Every building was razed to the ground." Metz itself had escaped major damage. "Street cars were buzzing up and down, streets were lighted with gas or electric lights, store windows charmingly decorated and stores full of articles of all kinds resembling very much our modern American stores." The citizens of Metz were "cold and less friendly to Americans and spoke the German language almost exclusively."

Dyer and his friend returned to Belleville where on the night of December 15 two passenger trains collided in dense fog. One of the trains carried French soldiers who were returning home. Some had served at the front since the outbreak of hostilities. Dyer and his medical team established an aid-station to care for the injured and dying. They spent the next several hours bandaging wounds, splinting fractures, and treating dislocations, while rescuers sought to free numerous soldiers who had been trapped in the wreckage.

On December 18 the medical detachment marched eighteen miles through snow and freezing rain to Liverdun where they were billeted in filthy, lice-infested barracks. Subsequent orders directed them to an abandoned evacuation hospital. The ramshackle structure had dirt floors and no heating. The unit next marched through ice and snow to Moran where they entrained to Domfront, reaching that city on Christmas Eve. Dyer and the other medical officers stood in a freezing rain for hours, awaiting the return of a white billeting officer who had forgotten about them. Dyer wrote, "The truth of a text came to me. 'Foxes have holes and the fowls of the air have nests, but the Son of Man hath nowhere to lay his head.'" The unit would remain at Domfront for a month.

"The people of Domfront were extremely pleasant to us and showed us the greatest hospitality." Learning that W.E.B. DuBois was visiting the area, Dyer and his mates of the Medical Core invited the renowned writer, lecturer, and civil rights advocate to join them for dinner at a café. DuBois declined the officers' invitation to speak, stating that he had to abide by strict censorship. He promised his countrymen that "he would have plenty to say when he returned to the United States."

Several days later, Dr. Dyer fell victim to the dreaded influenza epidemic that would kill thousands of soldiers and civilians across Europe. Hospitalized for a week, he attributed his survival to the devoted care of his fellow physicians. Desperately weak, he accompanied his unit to Le Mans where the soldiers would be processed through the Army's delousing station. Dyer sustained severe frostbite of his feet during the journey, but careful treatment by his medical comrades prevented the loss of toes.

The 317th Ammunition Train moved to Brest to prepare for embarkation to the States. During previous journeys by train, Dr. Dyer and the other officers rode in Pullman cars, while enlisted men traveled in freight cars. Orders for the trip to Brest specified that black officers would be allowed to travel only in the overcrowded freight cars. Intense cold greeted Dr. Dyer at Brest. Officers and men shared long wooden barracks. A wood stove at either end provided inadequate heat. The soldiers collected wood for small stoves that they added to the cubicles of the barracks. One day a white general arrived and ordered the removal of all the stoves. In the ensuing intense cold many soldiers contracted influenza, and several men died. Racial hazing had not ceased at war's end.

The much-anticipated march to the docks began on February 22, 1919. Before it began, the officers and men were warned that any soldier making "an unfavorable appearance" would be detained indefinitely in France. The march reminded Dyer "more of a funeral procession."

The troops sailed on the *Aquitania,* reaching New York City on February 28. Administrative duties took the group to Camp Dix, New

Jersey. On March 5, Dr. Dyer received a letter of commendation from his commanding officer, Major M.T. Dean. The letter spoke of the doctor's "manly qualities." The Major wrote, "I have always found you to be most efficient, dependable, conscientious in the performance of your duties and exacting in requiring those under you to zealously carry out instructions. Your efficient service has contributed to dispel the assertion of many that the Colored officer did not possess the qualities required in a commander of troops." I have not been able to establish the race of the Major.

"March 23rd my orders came and about noon I received my Honorable Discharge, which ended my service with Uncle Sam's Army."

I cannot yet close a thirty-nine-year gap in the life of Dr. Dyer. From William Maxwell's story and from an obituary in the Lincoln newspaper of January 22, 1958, I learned that Dyer had resumed his medical practice in Kansas City, Kansas. He served as a surgeon for the Santa Fe Railroad and for the Kansas City Police Department. I presume that he was assigned to the care of African American employees of the two agencies. Two years before his death, Lincoln College honored him at a banquet for distinguished alumni.

Billie Dyer died of a heart attack while driving one evening in Kansas City and was buried in Lincoln. Bessie Bradley Dyer survived him by one year. They had no children. In Lincoln's Old City Cemetery the top line of their shared headstone reads "DYER," beneath which were two engraved rectangles. The left reads "Bessie L. 1889-1959." The right reads "Dr. William H. 1886-1958."

Accompanying my copy of Dr. Dyer's diary were two letters from him to friends Hugh and Esther Davis. The handwriting was remarkably legible and identical to that of the diary. A letter dated November 17, 1957 reported an exhausting schedule due to an epidemic of Asian flu. The writer commented upon the launch of Sputnik, world and national politics, and Bessie's palpitations. He anticipated a reunion and refresher course sponsored by the Medical Alumni of the University of Illinois. He closed the letter: "I am, Your friend, Billie." Dyer sent a second letter from Chicago to his friends. After viewing the expansion of the University, he concluded, "As I looked around at the great improvements, I realized that I was born just fifty years too soon." The letters document Dr. Dyer's continuing, close observation of his environment, his abiding interest in history, and his commitment to medical practice. Age had not dimmed any of his faculties. He cherished his friends and medical associates and maintained a full-time medical practice until the time of his death.

Despite pursuing several leads, I could not locate any colleagues or former patients of Dr. Dyer either in Lincoln, Illinois or Kansas City, Kansas. I presume from the professional attitude which the diary so amply documents that Billie Dyer rendered expert, compassionate care to all of his civilian patients.

★　★　★

Billie Dyer's diary raises disturbing issues of covert and blatant racism in the US Army during World War I. While white combat units mobilized, trained, and embarked for western Europe, the black soldiers of the 92nd Division maintained a dreary routine of drill and classroom study. Dyer never alluded to the content of the classes. Nine months would elapse between his departure from Lincoln and his sailing from Trenton. Units of the 92nd Division in varying stages of preparedness would trickle across the Atlantic over a span of four months. Someone in higher military authority had decided to make the division irrelevant to the outcome of the war. I presume that political pressure led to the formation of the division, but this pressure could not influence what the Army actually did with the division once it assembled at military camps.

American troops were urgently needed at the battlefront. White troops entered the combat zone within weeks of enlistment. In 1960 I met in Lebanon, Illinois a veteran of World War I, a white, retired farmer. In a conversation after dinner he described his own induction into military service in 1917. He was assigned to an infantry battalion. The inductees received little instruction other than how to wear their uniforms and how to march. Trains brought them to New York City. Accompanied by other newly formed combat units, they marched through Manhattan to the docks, cheered along the way by flag-waving crowds. He recalled being warned by his commanding officer that any soldier attempting to break ranks and flee would be shot on the spot.

Training for combat began aboard ship and continued after disembarking in France. Within a few days of their arrival in Europe the white units marched into combat.

In the meantime, the separated units of the 92nd Division moved from one French town to another, sometimes by train, sometimes by truck, sometimes afoot. Typically, Billie and his team would arrive at an assigned destination, usually a dirty, long-abandoned barracks. After unpacking their gear and cleaning the premises, they would receive fresh orders directing them to another town. Sometimes the 317th Ammunitions Train would spend weeks in a town with no orders except to drill. The officers wondered at times if their unit had simply been forgotten. Those in command of American forces seemed to have one overriding goal in regard to the 92nd Division: prevent its contact with any white troops.

The Battle of Metz marked the 92nd Division's first chance to fight at full strength. Smaller units had participated in skirmishes earlier in the war. The 92nd acquitted itself with distinction in two days of intense fighting. The reasons for attacking Metz remain unclear. The German forces surrounding the city presented no threat to Allied forces. Negotiations for an armistice were well under way at the time of the battle. While action paused in other sectors, the 92nd engaged in some of the fiercest fighting of the war. Possibly a black commander saw Metz as an opportunity to prove the combat-worthiness of his men. Alternatively, a white commander may have viewed Metz as a place where the black division might be bloodied in a campaign that had no strategic value.

The patience and composure exhibited by Dr. Dyer throughout his year and a half of Army service strains credulity. He endured shabby billets, including a stable at his first posting. He read orders aboard the ship bound for Europe that reinstituted segregationist practices of the American South. He mourned the "lynching" of a young black private. He read with amazement the official document that directed black soldiers to handle victims of mustard gas. He endured freezing temperatures after a white officer removed the stoves from his barracks. In his diary Billie never gave way to rage. Racial affronts evoked sorrow and disappointment in his fellow white soldiers. He never expressed regret that he had enlisted in the Army of the United States.

Doctor Dyer found gratitude and acceptance by French civilians at all levels of society. Evenings spent over dinner in French homes gave him lasting images of what could be achieved in a society with no racial barriers. With ease he could teach rudiments of English to his French hosts while they helped him with his French vocabulary and accent. He did not discuss the politics and customs of the United States with his French acquaintances. He repeatedly noted the burdens borne by the French people. He lamented the ruined villages with their burned churches and shell-pocked fields. He mourned the French soldiers who were buried by the thousands in the countryside through which he passed, and his compassion extended to the dead of the German Air Force. His generous spirit harbored no animosity.

A picture finally emerges from the diary of a volunteer soldier devoted to the principles of democracy even if his homeland continued to struggle with the concept of equality for all its citizens. Billie Dyer, the physician, served wherever and whenever sick or wounded people needed help. He moved smoothly and expertly from dispensary to meningitis ward to sites of mass trauma. His love and enthusiasm for his work shows in his diary and in the two letters written in the year before his death. He cherished Bessie from the days of courtship in Kansas City until his life's end.

The question continues for me, "How did he do it?" A fresh insight came from a patient and friend of thirty years. James Towns, an African American retiree from a candy company, and I share a hometown — LaGrange, Georgia. Our experiences there, however, were radically different. I spent my boyhood on the white side of the segregationist barrier. I had ready access to a municipal swimming pool, a public library, and a cinema. I was free to go wherever I pleased in the business district and white residential neighborhoods. James Towns knew the same town as a place of unpaved streets, shabby housing, and no public amenities. He had limited access to the shopping and business district and only then if an adult accompanied him.

We have entirely different but surprisingly happy memories of our childhood and teen years. James Towns attends a yearly reunion in our hometown. During a visit in the summer of 2003, I asked him how he had sustained his gentle, good nature in a setting of rigid racial and economic segregation. He paused before replying, "I had good parents. They taught me never to let anger control me. If someone mistreated me, I was to pray for them." I had my breakthrough into the character of Billie Dyer.

I have further work to do. Surely, there is a surviving patient in Kansas City or a record of his work with the Santa Fe Railroad or the Kansas City police department. Perhaps the transcript of his studies at the University of Illinois will turn up. I will leave flowers when next I visit his grave.

SOURCES AND ACKNOWLEDGMENTS

William Maxwell's story launched my enquiry. Richard Sumrall, Director of the Lincoln Public Library, provided me with a copy of Billie Dyer's diary. Debbie Ackerman welcomed me to Lincoln College and located his undergraduate transcript. Staff at the Special Collections Department, Library of the Health Sciences, University of Illinois at Chicago located a photograph of Dr. Dyer taken in 1916. Gail Buckley's *American Patriots: The Story of Blacks in the Military from the Revolution to Desert Storm* (2001) provided invaluable insights into the history of black servicemen. James Towns' friendship has brightened many of my days.

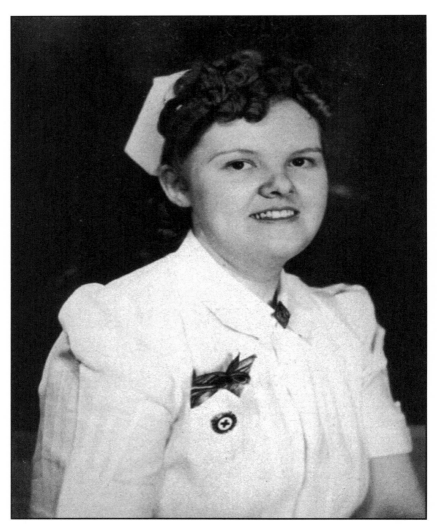

Vera Gustafson, RN

TWO NEW FEET: THE WORLD WAR II EXPERIENCES OF VERA GUSTAFSON

The right wheel squeaks ever so slightly as she maneuvers her wheelchair down the long hallway. She negotiates a sharp turn before backing her chair into the cramped examining room. Vera Palmer's rounded face seems to have but one expression, that of abiding optimism. During the twenty-five years of our acquaintance, her countenance has not seemed to age. Not so her knees. For years Vera has battled arthritis. Knee replacements have provided temporary relief from pain and immobility, but even new knees cannot compensate for hips and ankles that have seen too many miles. Diabetes and circulatory problems have taken further tolls upon her body, but her expression has remained unperturbed.

I learned during her initial visit to my office that she was a retired nurse and that she served in the United States Army during World War II. Vera volunteered nothing further. I did not press her for additional information. We had many other issues to address. During subsequent visits she made occasional reference to forthcoming reunions of her military unit, and from her equally taciturn husband, Walter, I learned that Vera and he had been assigned to the same evacuation hospital in Europe.

Perhaps we were both shaken by the tragedies of September 11, 2001. Perhaps Vera felt that it was time to unburden her memory. Or maybe we sought comfort and guidance from past experiences. Whatever our motivation, Vera and I scheduled the first of two lengthy chats about her experiences during World War II. We agreed upon a Saturday afternoon at her home in Red Bank, Tennessee. Vera greeted me from her lift-chair. Examples of her collection of knee-high, plaster elves adorned her living room. She had organized her scrapbooks, official military reports, snapshots, and letters for our discussion. We began, and I asked an occasional question or sought to clarify a point, but for the most part I listened while Vera related in sequence her experiences as Lieutenant Vera Gustafson. From time to time, she passed to me a photograph or official document to illustrate a certain memory.

Vera Gustafson's parents, Swan Joshua and Sophia, married in Chicago, the city to which they had immigrated from Sweden. Vera Doris Cecilia, their sixth daughter, was born on Saint Patrick's Day in 1917, and the subsequent birth of Swan Edward would complete the family. After her father's death when Vera was eight, the family endured protracted difficult times. Despite best efforts of the adult children who worked at various jobs, the Gustafsons lost their home to creditors, and the family had to move into cramped, rented housing. A sister, Ingabord, developed tuberculosis for which she required months in a sanatorium. "For awhile, the Church kept us afloat," Vera recalls.

After graduation from Austin High School, Vera pursued a long-held dream of becoming a registered nurse. That inspiration came from her cousin, Cecilia, who had served as a nurse during World War I. Cecilia provided the $400 needed to finance Vera's training, and after three years of intensive preparation, Vera received her nurse's cap from Augustana Swedish Lutheran Hospital in Chicago in 1939.

In a city still recovering from the Great Depression, jobs proved difficult to find. After a long and determined search, Vera obtained her first job in a clinic of five physicians. In addition to the duties of a nurse, she took dictation and performed the laboratory work for the practice. Attracted by better wages and working conditions, she accepted one year later the position of industrial nurse in the processing department of the Eastman Kodak Company. At Eastman, Vera manned a clinic for employees. Most of her patients suffered from skin rashes caused by chemicals used in the processing of color film. Pay was good, the hours regular. Vera, however, longed for something else, something that would capture the excitement that she had experienced on the clinical wards during her years of training. World War II would provide that opportunity.

As America recovered from the initial setbacks in the early months of the war, plans proceeded for an extended offensive campaign. Rapidly expanding armed forces would need a new and comprehensive system of hospitals to handle anticipated casualties. Medical centers across the United States formed military hospital units, recruiting physicians, nurses, and technical personnel for service. In the autumn of 1942, physicians from Augustiana, Swedish and Lutheran Hospital formed the nucleus of an evacuation hospital. This type of facility would triage and provide care for evacuees from frontline aid stations. The physicians sought additional recruits among current and former staff members and students who were young enough to enter active military duty and who were respected for their skills. Among the three hundred ten responders were fifty-two physicians and surgeons and forty-nine registered nurses, including Vera Gustafson.

Swan and Sophia had imbued Vera and her siblings with a deep sense of patriotism, and Vera desired much more clinical responsibility than her

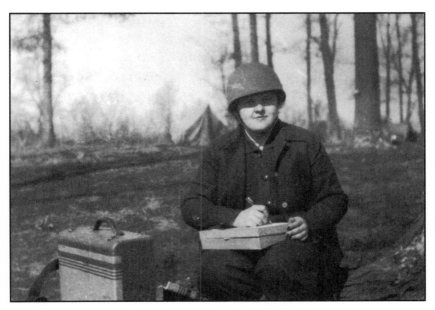

Second Lieutenant Vera Gustafson.

current job allowed. She also had a third motive for responding to the call for volunteers. Her brother Eddie had joined the Army Air Force soon after the attack on Pearl Harbor and, after flight training, received orders for Europe. Mother Sophia immediately despaired for Eddie's safety overseas but seemed reassured when she learned that Vera would serve in Europe as well. Vera promised to look after Eddie.

Vera took her oath of allegiance in October 1942 and entered the Army Nurses' Corps as a Second Lieutenant. She would be known as "Gussie" throughout her military career. I will employ her nickname for this chapter of her life.

Gussie's unit, the 27th Evacuation Hospital, spent the next 18 months in the United States, first at Camp Breckinridge, Kentucky in training with the Second Army. Obstacle courses and endurance marches competed with countless drills in setting up, taking down, and moving the mobile, tented evacuation hospital. In the hospital Vera wore a white uniform and nurse's cap. In the field she donned a steel helmet and blue slacks. Nurses had to purchase their own slacks because an official uniform for duty in combat had not yet been designed. The unit moved to Gallatin, Tennessee where Gussie encountered her first military casualties among paratroopers injured in practice jumps. Rigorous training continued during a wintertime posting to Elkins, West Virginia. The group prepared for a winter campaign in Europe as they cared for soldiers injured in mountain maneuvers. Gussie recalled the challenge of staying warm in tents half-buried in the snow. Troops dubbed the area "Pneumonia Valley."

In the spring of 1944, the members of the 27th Hospital, now expert in the rapid deployment of a complete field hospital in varied terrain and weather conditions, continued to train at Fort Devons, Massachusetts. Uniforms finally arrived for the nurses. The unit anxiously awaited orders to embark for Europe. These came in April. The officers and nurses of the 27th joined five thousand troops aboard the *USS Billy Mitchell,* which sailed, unescorted by combat vessels, from Newport News, Virginia. Nine quiet days later the troopship reached Casablanca, a city in which squalor and magnificent palaces existed side by side. The clinical team boarded windowless train cars for the journey to Oran. There the support staff, who had crossed the Atlantic Ocean as part of a convoy, rejoined them. In Oran Gussie and her colleagues dealt with the paradox of living in tents while receiving their meals in an elegant villa. The pause would be short, for Italy beckoned.

The Fifth Army had landed at Salerno, south of Naples, in September 1943. The Allied force included elements from France, French North African territories, Poland, India, and New Zealand. Fierce, sustained fighting against German forces produced heavy casualties and little headway in a campaign that had been designed to ease pressure on the Russian front and to reduce German forces in France. A second landing of Allied forces in January 1944 at Anzio failed to break the costly stalemate. Casualties steadily increased. Additional medical facilities were urgently needed. The 27th Evacuation Hospital awaited its first challenge in combat.

The *USHS Seminole* transported Gussie's unit to Naples, a journey of three days. Vera recalls the shock of seeing wrecked and smoldering Allied ships cluttering the harbor. Shoreline buildings had been bombed to rubble. Members of the medical team directed the swift unloading of the crates that contained all of the elements of their hospital. Officers, physicians, and nurses spent their first night ashore at Terme, a deserted, glass-roofed mineral spa once frequented by Mussolini. At midnight, air-raid sirens announced an attack. Gussie and the other members of the clinical staff donned their steel helmets as they huddled in the one room that had sound walls and a masonry ceiling. Nearby bomb blasts blew out all of the spa's windows. But the 27th sustained no casualties in its introduction to combat.

The next day the 27th erected the tents and prefabricated wards that would house a fifteen hundred-bed medical and surgical hospital. The fierce battle of nearby Monte Cassino raged. Repeated Allied assaults on the German forces occupying the bomb-ravaged site of an ancient monastery generated thousands of casualties for the newly established hospital. The 27th would remain in place for ten grueling weeks without a day of rest. The demanding days of stateside training seemed tame in comparison to the daily onslaughts of the wounded. In addition to American GIs, Arab soldiers and French Foreign Legionnaires received treatment in the increasingly efficient facility.

From the hospital's first deployment onward, Gussie served as a nurse in the shock tent, the triage point for the most severely wounded soldiers. Two or three nurses, a doctor, and several aides manned the shock unit. Casualties typically received first aid at battalion aid stations before being transported to the evacuation hospital. Badly wounded soldiers appeared on foot, or litter bearers brought them directly to the hospital. Nurses in the shock tent took vital signs, cleaned wounds, and administered intravenous infusions of plasma and penicillin while the triage physician determined the extent of wounds. Within minutes the wounded soldier would be on his way by stretcher to the surgical tent, to an intensive care tent, or to one of the thirty-bed wards. Many soldiers died in the shock tent. Sometimes the streams of casualties seemed unending, and the planned, twelve-hour shifts had to overlap to cope with the numbers of patients. Once patients of the evacuation hospital achieved a stable status, ambulances transported them to a general hospital for further care.

Vera remembers the gratitude of the wounded French Foreign Legionnaires and colonial soldiers whom her unit treated. She remembers the name — Ben Saalem — of a seven-foot-tall North African soldier with multiple gunshot wounds to his shoulder and thigh and recalls that he recovered fully. A snapshot from that time shows Gussie

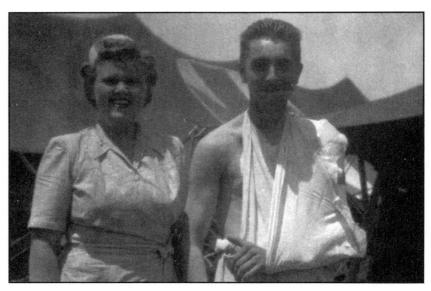

Nurse Vera Gustafson with a wounded soldier.

in her war-zone uniform, a brown and white striped seersucker dress, as she stands among a multinational group of recovering warriors, a stunning portrayal of order and cleanliness amid the grime and gore of war. "Exhaustion was not a problem in Italy," Vera recalls. "We had too much important work to do."

As action along the western coast of Italy subsided, Gussie joined a small group of colleagues in a brief and unofficial trip to Rome. Declared AWOL, the band of tourists received formal reprimands and restriction to their base. "We were restricted to where we spent all of our time anyway."

Its work completed in Italy, the 27th Evacuation Hospital packed its gear and sailed aboard *USHS Acadia* to join the Seventh Army. Just before her departure from Italy, Gussie learned that brother Eddie, copilot of a B-24 heavy bomber, had perished when his aircraft was brought down by enemy fire over Germany. Gussie felt that she had failed both her mother and her brother, but new orders precluded mourning. The memory of Eddie's loss still cuts deeply.

The Seventh Army had invaded France at Marseilles and attacked northward. Strategists hoped that this action would relieve pressure on Allied forces that landed in Normandy. Once a perimeter had been established, the 27th moved ashore, landing at St. Tropez. Gussie shouldered her pack as she climbed down rope ladders to the landing craft that would take her team to the beach. Trucks and ambulances carried the hospital unit to Aix-en-Provence where French citizens showered them with fruit and freshly baked bread.

In three hours, the hospital team was able to set up their seven hundred fifty-bed hospital — receiving ward, operating and recovery tents, wards, laboratory, and tents and kitchen facilities for patients and staff — and begin processing casualties. When the battlefront moved, the hospital quickly followed, tents and equipment to crates, crates to trucks, staff to trucks and jeeps. The cycle of set-up and take-down of the hospital would be repeated many times with few glitches. Sometimes the wounded arrived before a complete hospital could be erected. Treatment began with or without a canvas cover.

When the 27th reached Aix-en-Provence, casualties were already lined up. At this site the hospital would care for American, French and British soldiers, French civilians, and members of the French Resistance. Fatigue slowly mounted in the face of unceasing arrivals at the shock tent, but morale never faltered.

Vera pauses to recall an eighteen-year-old French male civilian with a closed fracture of his thigh. Policy dictated that once stabilized, French civilians should be sent to nearby civilian hospitals. The Army surgeons set the fracture and placed the leg in traction before transferring the young man to the closest community hospital. When aides traveled several days later to the French hospital to collect the traction apparatus, they learned that the boy's leg had been amputated. Upon learning this, Gussie and her nurse colleagues vowed never again to transfer anyone to a local hospital. Unfortunately, the French facilities lacked both supplies and experienced clinical staff.

A few days later, an eight-year-old French boy arrived at the shock tent. While his family sought shelter from a firefight, the boy's father had stepped on an anti-personnel mine. The blast killed the man instantly. His wife suffered serious wounds to her legs and abdomen, and her son sustained a severe wound to his hand. Rather than transfer the boy, Gussie and her nurse colleagues hid him while nursing him back to health. Once his wound had healed, the boy was discharged to the care of family members with both hands intact.

Within a month of setting up a hospital at Aix, the 27th dismantled their facility to move in the footsteps of the rapidly advancing Seventh Army. They traveled northward by train and truck to reach the town of Xertigny during the night of October 29. Their equipment arrived the next day, and by that evening the 27th Evacuation Hospital was back in full operation. During a month of almost constant rain the hospital treated ten thousand patients.

As the Seventh Army drove steadily northwards into the Vosges Mountains of northeastern France, casualties continued unabated. Wounded soldiers and civilians arrived at the evacuation hospital by field ambulance, jeep, and sometimes stretchers that seemed to appear from nowhere. Soldiers with appalling wounds might stagger into the shock tent under their own power. With speed and precision the team at the shock tent, working without a break, evaluated, stabilized, and readied their patients for the next level of care. Casualty lists at that time show open fractures, shrapnel, bullet, and blast wounds to head, thorax, groin, and extremities. Neither wounds nor care for these wounds relented.

Torrential rains turned the landscape at Xertigny into ankle-deep mud. Once in the middle of an abdominal surgery on a severely wounded GI, the tent covering the operating suite collapsed. Nurses and aides supported the sodden canvas until the surgeon, Dr. Lundgren, could complete the procedure. The soldier survived, and in a remarkable set of coincidences convalesced in a military hospital in Galesburg, Illinois where a volunteer involved in his care turned out to be a Mrs. Lundgren, mother of the surgeon.

As the Seventh Army resumed its advance, the 27th Evacuation Hospital relocated to nearby Baccarat where the hospital could establish itself in bomb-damaged buildings that featured wood-burning stoves and running water, luxuries for Gussie and her comrades. Twenty-two hundred and fifty patients proceeded through the shock tent and into the hospital at Baccarat during a four-week stay. Official reports document complex and frequently multiple wounds to every organ system of the body. "Multiple gunshot wounds to thorax." "Shrapnel wound to pelvis." "Open fracture of left femur." Nurses and doctors worked swiftly in teams to sustain life in bodies so cruelly damaged. Reading the stark clinical reports of the 27th Evacuation Hospital, I am reminded of a quotation attributed to Sir Richard Doll: "Statistics are people with the tears wiped away." I wondered about the subsequent lives of the young men who survived their wounds. In addition to the wounded, the hospital treated numerous medical patients who suffered from pneumonia, hepatitis, skin infections, and dysentery.

In late December 1944, during the chaos and uncertainty of a massive German counterattack — the Battle of the Bulge — the hospital moved to the village of Hagenau, only five miles from the German border. The staff returned to their customary tents. Brutally cold weather dictated that the nurses swap their smocks for woolen trousers and shirts.

At Hagenau, Gussie fell in love. Before leaving Oran in North Africa, she had been introduced to Sergeant Walter Palmer who served as the butcher for the hospital's kitchen. In the frozen setting of Hagenau, Sergeant Palmer became Patient Palmer, felled abruptly by a high fever and severe headache. Studies proved inconclusive. Walter's physicians considered widespread tuberculosis and viral encephalitis as possible diagnoses. Neither could be treated at the evacuation hospital. An ambulance took Sergeant Palmer to a general hospital on the French-Swiss border where his condition remained precarious. Gussie hitched a ride in an ambulance to visit Walter. His physician described Gussie as "a vision from Heaven, just what Walter needs."

Although his weight had fallen to eighty pounds, Walter rallied, and soon he received fresh orders. Through a mix-up, however, Walter found himself in the wrong replacement depot. Fearing that he would lose Gussie, Walter commandeered at pistol-point an ambulance to return him to his unit. There his colonel "adjusted" the orders of the 27th's cherished butcher so that he could remain with them. Vera recalls, "I couldn't help it that I fell in love with stripes on his sleeve and not chickens (the eagles on the epaulets of colonels) on his shoulder."

Later in the stay at Hagenau, the still-thin Walter would surprise Gussie with an invitation to join him for breakfast in his tent. The butcher had sole occupancy of a large tent in which he would cut and prepare meat for the hospital. Atop a wooden trunk, Walter spread platters of eggs, bacon, and fresh strawberries. Just then, Gussie's commanding officer appeared at the entrance to Walter's tent, shook her head in disbelief and walked away. The strict prohibition of dating between officers and non-commissioned officers obviously had eased.

The hospital in Hagenau lay between a busy railroad on one side and an airfield on the other. Artillery of the opposing armies continually whined overhead. "We learned not to pay any attention to it. No one was hurt." Once a reconnaissance vehicle arrived. Rumors had reached Seventh Army headquarters that the evacuation hospital had been annihilated, and the vehicle had been dispatched to determine if the facility had been lost. Gussie and her team assured the driver that she and her colleagues were alive and fully functional.

During a brief lull on Christmas Day 1944 Gussie and several nurses accepted an invitation for dinner in the home of a French family. A simple, hot meal, elegantly served, reminded Gussie of earlier Christmas dinners in her Chicago home.

As the American forces beat back German forces in the Vosges

Mountains, work intensified for the 27th. Early in January Gussie was astonished by the arrival of wounded Japanese soldiers in American uniforms. These troops were members of the famed 442nd Regimental Combat Team composed of Japanese-American volunteers, many recruited from detention camps in the United States. This unit received more citations for valor than any other during World War II. Their unit had sustained heavy casualties in rescuing an encircled battalion of paratroopers, the famed "Lost Battalion" of the Vosges Mountains.

At this point in Vera's narration of her story, we pause. Vera's eyes fill with tears as she recalls a young Japanese-American soldier. "His name was Danny. He had been shot to hell. He had a bad head wound. He was conscious at first. We knew he would not make it."

Gussie cradled the soldier's head in one arm while she slowly administered intravenous medication with the other. The triage physician asked to relieve Gussie and continued the medication until the soldier died.

Among many emotional traumas, the most severe befell Gussie during her assignment in Hagenau. During a rainy night a US truck collided with a civilian vehicle. French civilians and a badly injured GI arrived by ambulance at the shock tent. Determining that the GI was Roman Catholic, Gussie sent for a chaplain of his faith. The nearest Catholic chaplain was assigned to a nearby Air Force group. En route to the evacuation hospital the chaplain's jeep crashed into a truck, and the chaplain died at the scene. Upon learning of this death, the Captain officer-of-the-day "bawled me out for calling for the chaplain and causing his death. My heart was broken." When her shift ended, Gussie requested permission to accompany another chaplain on the jeep ride to his base. Tears overwhelmed her. "You did what you were supposed to do, Lieutenant," the chaplain gently counseled her.

For its actions during this chapter of the war, the 27th received a Citation of Merit, and Gussie was promoted to First Lieutenant. The evacuation hospital returned to Baccarat, this time for eleven weeks, during which six thousand casualties received care from the clinical team.

Finally, hostilities slowed sufficiently that nurses in small groups could undertake weekend furloughs, their first in Europe. Gussie and several friends arranged passage to London. The British capital, however, was anything but safe. Several times each day V-1 rockets screeched across the sky before crashing into random targets on the ground. Gussie somehow managed to tune out fear while concentrating upon the sights of the city. After London the nurses traveled to Salisbury where Gussie found a special serenity inside and around the famed Cathedral. When they returned to duty, the nurses attended Easter services at the American Cathedral in Paris.

The Seventh Army fought its way across the Rhine River into Germany. The 27th raised its tents outside the town of Goldheim before moving to Hosbach where an ambulance brought a pregnant German woman to the hospital. She had a severe head injury for which little could be done, but the surgeon delivered a healthy baby boy by Caesarian section before his mother died, and the baby was transferred to a German hospital.

No one could have anticipated the next challenge for the doctors and nurses of the evacuation hospital. On March 30, 1945, ambulances began a shuttle of American prisoners of war freed from a nearby camp. Two hundred POWs received care before evacuation to France. ("They were so pitiful, so emaciated," Vera remembers.) They described a commandant who had a special hatred of Americans. While prisoners of other nationalities received subsistence diets, Americans were limited to two hundred calories per day. Several of the newly freed men died at the evacuation hospital. Many had severe tuberculosis. All seemed emotionally devastated.

One ambulance unloaded a thin young POW who held tightly to a blanket covering his abdomen and legs. Gussie tried to bathe him, but the soldier refused her pleas to remove his blanket. After a brief stand-off, the young man jerked the blanket from his body, declaring "See, no feet!"

"You weren't supposed to show emotion," Vera recalls. "We were to do our job." Fixing the young soldier's eyes with her own, she promised, "We'll get you back to the States and get you some fine, new feet." And then she finished bathing her patient.

Sergeant Palmer appeared with steaks for the newly freed men. The colonel protested. "Palmer you can't give steak to these men. You'll kill them." "Colonel, if I can't do it, then you do it," the butcher replied as he handed a fork to the officer. Walter repeatedly took stands on behalf of hungry soldiers and civilians. The colonel paused for a moment as he looked at the faces of men who stared at the sizzling steaks. "Okay, Palmer. Do the best you can."

The Seventh Army entered Bavaria, and the hospital set up its tents on the grounds of a horse breeding farm at Starnberg near Munich. "The country was so beautiful so different from where we had been," Vera remembers.

One day, at an urgently convened meeting of the hospital's staff, the colonel called for volunteers to embark on a short-term assignment. The concentration camp at Dachau had just been liberated. Medical care was desperately needed for the survivors. Ten nurses, several doctors, and their supporting staff would comprise the detachment from the 27th Evacuation Hospital. Gussie was one of many who stepped forward. The volunteers, not knowing what to expect, quickly loaded medications, intravenous fluids, and surgical dressings into the trucks and jeeps that would take them to the camp.

Dachau's infamy dated from its construction in 1933. It would serve as a model for later concentration camps, and personnel destined for other camps received their training there. Jews, Gypsies, and political opponents of Hitler were placed in the camp, and untold thousands perished from starvation, disease, and execution at the hands of the Nazis. After processing at Dachau, hundreds of thousands of prisoners were shipped to extermination camps.

The small convoy arrived at a scene of utter desolation. Several hundred inmates, "the "living dead," clung to life. Troops from the 442nd Regimental Combat Team had broken the padlocks on the camp, and the liberating soldiers had done all that was possible with their limited resources to alleviate the suffering at the camp. Burial teams coped with stacks of corpses, and Gussie and her team would spend ten days establishing a system of medical care. The routine was the same as that of the shock tent: clean, assess, dress wounds, stabilize, administer fluids and penicillin. But there was no place to which these patients could be transferred.

All of the surviving inmates were severely emaciated. Many had typhus. Few could stand or walk without assistance. Despite the efforts of the doctors and nurses, scores would die each day, too frail to respond to care. Gussie learned that the only medical therapy available to the inmates in the weeks before liberation had been at the hands of a carpenter who worked as a surgeon in the camp's dispensary.

Despite the widespread use of disinfectants, the omnipresent stench of death could not be eradicated. The most severely starved inmates received liquid diets. They assumed that they were being punished, unable to understand that their stomachs and intestines could not yet tolerate solid nourishment. Gussie observed that inmates strong enough to receive solid food routinely hid portions in their garments. She found macaroni and cheese sequestered in the bedclothes of prisoners when she made her morning rounds. Even after liberation, the former prisoners feared that food might abruptly and arbitrarily be taken away. The craving for food superseded all other needs.

Gussie could deal calmly and expertly with the wounds of combat, but she had never seen physical and mental wounds of the kind that she witnessed at Dachau. She and the members of her team could barely keep at bay a sense of hopelessness. Each day, however, lifted a few more of the former inmates to a higher level of self-care and independence.

Other medical units arrived. After ten exhausting days that would haunt Gussie forever, she and the detachment of volunteers returned to their hospital. A blurred snapshot from this mission shows the wraith-like figure of a prisoner in a ragged, striped uniform. He stands behind barbed wire. He stares passively at the camera. Would he live beyond that day?

The hospital moved to Darmstadt, and Gussie and several nursing colleagues established contact with civilians in the wrecked city. They paid German women to do their laundry and gave small tips to German children as rewards for errands. Walter Palmer and a companion accepted an invitation for coffee at the home of a boy whom they had befriended, and they learned that the coffee served by their hosts had been brewed from grounds scavenged from trash cans outside military mess halls. From then on Walter found ways to smuggle coffee and food to the hungry civilians. Vera and a nurse friend learned of a starved Lutheran minister who lay near death in his home. He had given his rations to children of his neighborhood. To the chagrin of a captain, Vera and the nurses provided vitamins and Walter found food for the clergyman. By the time of the hospital's departure the pastor had recovered sufficient strength to walk. Vera exchanges Christmas cards yearly with two of the German boys, now men, whom she met and befriended at Darmstadt.

Ever so slowly, the fighting subsided. German forces surrendered on May 8, 1945. Gussie and her colleagues entrained to Marseilles where she briefly saw at a distance the Aga Khan, and she arrived in New York City in November. After discharge from active duty, she returned to Chicago and her old job at Eastman Kodak. She now welcomed the slower pace and predictable routine. Walter Palmer soon came home as well. He had plans for his "angel." In June 1946 they married in St. Paul's Evangelical Lutheran Church.

Vera and Walter moved into a new house at 109 Forsythe Street in Red Bank, Tennessee where Vera resides to this day. Walter continued his work as a meat cutter for restaurants in Chattanooga, and Vera worked for a time as a nurse at the city's Erlanger Hospital, although after the births of two sons, Benny and Eddie, Vera reduced her nursing duties to part-time. Throughout the years, Vera and Walter attended several reunions of the 27th Evacuation Hospital.

After Walter, "the love of my life," died in 1993, and the further decline of her own health, Vera had to limit her contacts with her one-time Army colleagues to occasional letters and Christmas cards. During our interview, she had referred to her husband-to-be as Palmer. I asked her what she called him once they were married. "Sometimes 'Palmer,' but mostly 'Walter' or 'Dear,'" she answered.

Her story concluded, we sat quietly for a time, each of us reflecting upon the amazing and sorrowful and heroic times in which Vera had served her country. After our three-hour-long focus upon war, we spoke of the blessings of children and family and wondered how anyone could sink to levels of brutality such as Vera saw at Dachau. I contemplated the sheer numbers of casualties treated by Vera's hospital.

The outside light began to fade, and it was time for me to leave. Vera slowly pulled herself erect, leaned forward to support herself on her walker, and accompanied me to her front door.

Vera comes to my office at regular intervals for monitoring of her diabetes and her circulatory problems. The casual observer in the waiting room sees a bespectacled, white-haired lady, a bit overweight, pleasant in her dealings with staff at the front desk. I imagine Norman Rockwell selecting her to pose for a painting of the quintessential grandmother. There is no hint that informs employees and other patients that they are in the presence of a remarkable veteran of World War II, a nurse who at various times rendered care to grotesquely wounded soldiers, to tubercular POWs, to victims of the Holocaust. She could work nonstop when casualties piled up, sustaining with her coworkers in the shock tent a routine of precision, efficiency, and above all else, compassion.

A primary motive for enlisting, the safeguarding of her brother Eddie, ended in tragedy. Vera honors his memory and wonders what she could have done to protect him. When her mother and sisters sought Vera's opinion for relocating Eddie's remains from a cemetery in Europe to one in America, she convinced them that "Eddie should be allowed to rest where he is."

Vera's memories are quite precise; she recalls names, dates, and places with great clarity. As she recounted her story, I sensed that details and emotions that have been stored in separate files became reconnected. She maintains regular contact with her closest friend and tentmate, Ruth Schrader, nicknamed Ci. Their exchanges deal with the present, the state of their health, events in the lives of their families, and not with the shared and wrenching experiences with the evacuation hospital. War defined Vera, showing her quite explicitly that she could manage every conceivable challenge a nurse might encounter, but she does not dwell upon the events of wartime. Marriage and the building of a family became her guiding passions.

During a recent visit I opined, "Vera, I consider you a hero."

"No, I'm really not," she replied. "I just tried to do my job."

SOURCES AND ACKNOWLEDGMENTS

Delivered from Evil: The Saga of World War II (1987) by Robert Leckie provides a succinct overview of Allied actions in Italy, France, and Germany. *Monte Cassino: The Story of the Most Controversial Battle of World War II* (1984) by David Hapgood and David Richardson offers a detailed history of the pivotal battle in the Allies drive to Rome. Actions of the Seventh Army in the north of France are covered in *When the Odds Were Even: The Vosges Mountains Campaign, October 1944–January 1945* (1994) by Keith E. Bonn. *The Last Escape: The Untold Story of Allied Prisoners of War in Europe, 1944-45* (2002) by John Nichol and Tony Rennell offers fresh information. *The World Must Know: The History of the Holocaust as Told in the United States Holocaust Memorial Museum* (1993) by Michael Berenbaum presents with extensive photographs a passionate summary of Hitler's plans to exterminate the Jews of Europe.

IN TIMES
OF PEACE

—∿∿—

*There has to be something beautiful
beyond this.*

— HAT CHAU

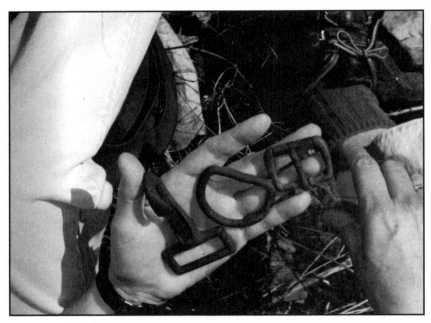

*Burned equipment left behind by the
smokejumpers in the Mann Gulch fire of 1949.*

A HIKE INTO MANN GULCH:
THE DEADLY FOREST FIRE
OF 1949

—⁓—

From the boat landing, Mann Gulch seemed well within my hiking capa-
bilities. Though close upon sixty, I considered myself reasonably fit. I
worked out at the YMCA regularly and could walk indefinitely in rolling
countryside. Initially I kept up with my wife and our young guide. Thirty
minutes into the hike, however, I struggled to get my breath and to keep
up with my companions who were now far ahead of me. I had misread
the steepness of the canyon walls, the effect of altitude, and the heat of a
late summer morning. Footing was treacherous in the knee-high grass.
But this hike was necessary, a chance to understand puzzles that dated
from boyhood. I had come to Mann Gulch because of a fascination with
smokejumpers and because of a book, *Young Men and Fire*, written by
Norman Maclean and published four years earlier.

Since childhood I have stood in awe of smokejumpers. The idea of
people actually parachuting into remote areas to fight forest fires struck
me as the height of bravery. Two books by Montgomery Atwater —
Hank Winton: Smokechaser and *The Forest Rangers* — fired my imagination and introduced me to this world of danger and high purpose. My
peers and I quickly adapted roles from these books into afternoon play,
using kudzu vines that dangled over a sawdust pit to simulate the lines
of parachutes that would safely guide us into imagined action.

My admiration for smokejumpers grew with the release of *Red Skies of Montana*. This 1952 movie starred Richard Widmark as the leader of a team of smokejumpers, many of whom perished when a fire exploded out of control. The film uniquely captured the awesome power and speed of the windblown inferno as it overtook, and killed, the firefighters. Widmark's character was charged with behaving recklessly and causing the death of his men. I later learned that the movie had been loosely based upon a real fire that had swept up a canyon, Mann Gulch, near Helena, Montana.

Occasional newspaper accounts of firefighters and the perils that they encountered stimulated anew my regard for these airborne forest rangers. In the 1980s I encountered a beguiling book, *A River Runs Through It and Other Stories*, by Norman Maclean. One of the novellas in the collection dealt with the experiences of a young forest ranger in 1919. Toughness, loyalty, and mutual esteem characterized the men of the crew. When *Young Men and Fire* appeared in 1992, I quickly purchased it. Within its pages I found a powerful narrative of young smokejumpers who had been destroyed by fire. I learned much about fire science and started understanding the drives and motives of young smokejumpers.

Young Men and Fire detailed the author's attempt of many years to untangle conflicting accounts of the tragedy at the deadly fire in Mann Gulch. Maclean, a retired professor of English literature at the University of Chicago, began his investigation when he was seventy-four years old. With the passion of a sleuth seeking clues to an unsolved mystery, he tracked down the two remaining survivors of the fire crew, examined all of the official proceedings that he could locate, and studied fire science extensively. Accompanied and aided throughout this endeavor by a veteran forest ranger and smokejumper, Laird Robinson, Maclean made repeated visits by horseback into the Mann Gulch. Upon his death in 1990 at age eighty-seven, Maclean left a manuscript for his editorial colleagues at the University of Chicago Press to complete and release in 1992.

The tragedy at Mann Gulch began on August 5, 1949. Fifteen smokejumpers had parachuted into the canyon to fight a fire begun by a random lightning strike during the previous day. The area had been suffering from record-high temperatures. The men parachuted in mid-afternoon onto a gentle slope at the head of the canyon and were joined on the ground by a forester from a nearby station. They had gathered their equipment and begun an orderly march toward the fire when suddenly the fire exploded into a fiery wind that charged ferociously towards them. The blaze cut off an escape route to the river. Discarding their packs and equipment, the men raced up canyon, through dry brush and waist-high grass. Their goal was the barren, rocky crest of the south wall of the canyon — they would be safe once they were at the ridgeline. Two men managed to outrun the fire and escape through a slit in overhanging rocks, but the crew chief, realizing that he could not outrun the fire, set a small fire in front of himself, lay down in its ashes, and survived as the main fire rushed over him. He screamed out instructions to his men to follow his example, but his words were lost in the noise of the conflagration.

Official hearings that followed the fire deemed the maneuver that saved his life to be an irresponsible act that had contributed to the deaths of thirteen of his men.

Norman Maclean visited the scene of the fire several days after the disaster. A native of Missoula, Montana, he knew fires well from his own experiences as a teenaged member of fire crews and had considered a career in the Forest Service. Through meticulous analysis and repeated on-site investigation, he established the sequence of events that took place during the Mann Gulch blaze. He determined the escape route of the two survivors who had outrun the fire as well as the location of the crew chief's "escape" fire. Significantly, his studies vindicated the actions of the crew chief and showed conclusively that the small fire which the chief had ignited did not cause or even contribute to any loss of life.

In his book Maclean contemplates the motives of young men who pursue dangerous endeavors. Events in his own life repeatedly intertwine with his "fire report," so that author and reader share a meditation on loss of youth and loss of loved ones. Throughout *Young Men and Fire* Maclean speaks of the need to change catastrophe to tragedy. Catastrophe seems random and inexplicable, negating bravery and destroying in one sweep human plans and aspirations, whereas tragedy raises the loss to a level that permits moral and intellectual comprehension.

My chance to visit Mann Gulch arose with an invitation to the annual meeting of the Montana Chapter of the American College of Physicians. Helena served as the host city. At a dinner on the evening before my visit to Mann Gulch, I had the special privilege of meeting Laird Robinson and learning firsthand of the investigations he shared with Norman Maclean. Both men had been driven to establish the facts of the long-ago tragedy. They were comrades on a mission.

Our hosts arranged our journey upriver to Mann Gulch for early the next morning. My wife, our guide, and I just fit into the motorized rubber boat. As we puttered against the gentle current of the Missouri River, we saw bald eagles completing their morning searches for food. White mountain goats fed at water's edge, oblivious to our passing craft. The sky was cloudless, and the day was already hot with no breath of wind. We tied in at a small dock at the opening of Mann Gulch upon the river and, using a detailed topographic map and an annotated map from *Young Men and Fire,* planned a walk up-canyon. The ill-fated fire crew of 1949 had been cut off from the safety of the river by a wall of flames that raced toward them: we would seek to duplicate the path of the fire crew as they began their race up a steep wall that lay to our left.

Clusters of evergreen dotted the canyon. Trunks of trees that had been burned in the great fire lay on both slopes. Their crowns pointed upslope, away from the explosive force of the fire that had brought them down. The fire that had initially seemed small and routine had exploded when cooler air from the river was sucked into the canyon, which was suddenly transformed into giant chimney. A gale-like wind had resulted and rushed toward the head of the canyon. As I walked through the parched yellow grass that reached to my knees, I could feel the speed and hear the sound of fire tearing though this tinder. Estimates placed the speed of the advancing flames at sixty miles per hour.

I came to one granite cross, then another, each marking the site where one of the thirteen victims had fallen, each bearing a metal nameplate of that firefighter. Two men, horribly burned, would be evacuated to a hospital in Helena where they died within a day. The thirteen crosses were well maintained by colleagues who regularly visited Mann Gulch.

The gradient became steeper. Footing over loose rock became trickier. A rocky overhang seemed to block any exit from the canyon. My wife and the guide had gained the crest and directed me to a narrow break in the barrier through which I could pull myself. This same passageway had been used by the two survivors in 1949. I was exhausted by my climb. I could feel the desperation of the young smokejumpers in the smoke and searing heat, running up a progressively steeper slope, searching for a route of escape in the rocky wall that seemed to seal the canyon. Unusual fitness and luck had allowed just two men to endure, a sudden, fortuitous burst of ingenuity having spared the life of their chief.

After a brief rest and a lot of water, we began our descent. Our guide pointed out remnants of wooden pack frames and hardware that lay where the smokejumpers had dumped them in their race with fire. Persistent arid conditions had preserved the artifacts. In a rocky recess our guide showed us a corroded flashlight and metal buckles worn by the men forty-seven years earlier. The blackened remnants of packs and equipment constituted a different memorial to the tragic day so long ago. We paused at the mouth of the canyon to examine our maps and compare them once again with the terrain we had just traversed. The lines on the topographic map could not begin to adequately portray how steep the slopes of the canyon's walls were, or how much of a challenge they must have posed for the smokejumpers.

As we discussed the men and their failed mission on our return downriver, we observed mountain goats on the slopes that bordered the river. En route we passed a larger boat destined for Mann Gulch, and I wondered what had attracted the thirty or so people on its decks. I suspect that they, too, had long-abiding questions about fires and the people who fought them.

When I first encountered smokejumpers in adolescent fiction and in film, I marveled at the raw courage of the men. Though I had never seen forest firefighters in action, I had on two occasions, once in Florida and once in Alaska, watched as fires rapidly spread through dense national forests. The fire in northern Florida extended along both sides of the highway my parents and I traveled. I remember quite well the tremendous heat generated by the blaze. Further along the highway we were passed by fire engines and tankers rushing to the scene of the torrent.

I can imagine smokejumpers selecting their jobs in the same way as young Marine recruits. Endowed with high energy and curiosity, they volunteer motivated by desire for adventure and service. They do not entertain thoughts of their own mortality. The forest rangers whom I have met over the years cherish the forests and mountains and valleys of their jurisdictions. They seem especially content in their work.

John Maclean continued his father's passion for sifting fact from fiction in two studies of wildfire, *Fire and Ashes* and *Fire on the Mountain*. Both books honor the bravery and dedication of firefighters while meticulously describing the reckless power of forest fires. Both books have allowed me to continue a personal study that began so many years ago.

My favorite patch of trees is a stand of giant virgin pine within the Voyageurs National Park along the Minnesota–Canada border. Twice while carrying a canoe and camping gear I have walked among those trees whose needles create a thick, soft carpet over the forest's floor. Only a small stretch of the imagination is needed to understand a young man or young woman who is determined to protect such treasure from the ravages of wildfire.

I will always salute these woodland warriors and Norman Maclean, who revealed their work to me with quiet passion and intellectual integrity.

SOURCES AND ACKNOWLEDGMENTS

Norman Maclean's *A River Runs Through It and Other Stories* (1976) and *Young Men and Fire* (1992) together provide invaluable information on Montana in the early and middle years of the twentieth century and on forest fires and the fire service. The latter title is a result of one man's dedication to establishing the truth behind a disaster. John Maclean's *Fire on the Mountain* (1999) combines engaging narrative with meticulous research in itsreport of a Colorado forest fire that killed fourteen smokejumpers in July 1994. His *Fire and Ashes* (2003) analyzes two additional fires and includes an interview with the sole survivor of the Mann Gulch fire. Two articles by Professor Alan Weltzien of the English Department of the University of Western Montana in *Western American Literature* gave me deeper insights into the remarkable career of Norman Maclean (The Two Lives of Norman Maclean and the Text of Fire in *YoungMen and Fire,* Volume 29, Number 1, May 1994, pages 3-11; and "Norman Maclean and Tragedy," Volume 30, Number 2, August 1995, pages 139-149).

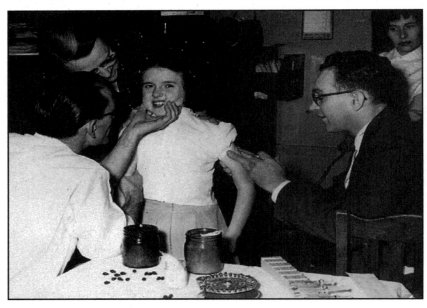

Dr. Woodrow Dodson immunizing a child.

LOCK AND DAM NUMBER 20:
WOODROW DODSON

—⁓⁓⁓—

The ring of the telephone interrupted supper. The caller reported that his wife's contractions had begun half an hour earlier. They were regular but unusually painful.

In ordinary times, Dr. Woodrow Dodson would have taken his delivery equipment and either driven across the bridge at Quincy or used the Canton ferry to cross to the Illinois side of the Mississippi. Once in his patient's home, he would have set up his portable delivery table, arranged his obstetrical tools, and waited with the family for the baby's crowning. Sometimes the wait in a patient's home would extend for half a night. As labor neared its conclusion, all but one female helper would leave the room until the completion of the delivery. The door would open and Dr. Dodson would announce the gender of the newborn. Typically, the father would then pay him the thirty-five-dollar delivery fee before the doctor returned home.

On this night, however, there was the blizzard. The ferry was out of service. Drifting snow made transfer of the patient to the hospital in Quincy impossible, and the doctor's automobile rested, inoperable, beneath a thick cover of snow and ice.

"I will be there shortly," he promised the caller. "Meet me at the dam."

Dr. Dodson, known as Woody to his friends and patients, checked his instruments before snapping shut his black bag. The collapsible delivery table fit snugly in its case with a sling that he placed upon his shoulder. Before setting out, he reassured his wife, Mary Jane, that he would phone once he reached his patient's home.

The mile-long walk to the dam presented the first challenge for Woody. Deep snow and a strong wind slowed his progress. Despite the cold, he perspired under his coat and woolen sweater. One step, and another and another; he broke a path to the river.

Lock and dam number 20 had been built years earlier for navigational and flood control purposes, part of an elaborate system of dams and levees erected by the US Army Corps of Engineers. The walkways across the lock and dam extended almost a mile to the Illinois shore. Ordinarily, no one would be permitted to make the walk across the revetment. Even in fair weather a misstep or a strong gust of wind could lead to serious injury, but Woody had explained his patient's dilemma to the lockmaster who reluctantly granted permission for the doctor to cross on foot.

Steeply pitched metal stairs led to the walkway over the lock. Once atop the lock, Woody searched for lights on the far shore, but the continuing snow blocked his view. Ever so slowly, watching the placement of each boot-step with his flashlight, he worked his way across the dam. Each of several lights along the walkway created a yellow-grey oasis toward which he would move. Reaching the far end of the dam, he carefully descended another metal stairway.

His patient's husband greeted him. The farmer had driven his tractor to the dam to meet the doctor. Woody knelt alongside the driver, who steered his tractor, retracing the trail of a mile and a half that he had cut through the snow. Finally they reached the farm house, its fencing hidden beneath the drifting snow. After his two-hour journey, Woody welcomed the warmth of the living room. Two women from a neighboring farm greeted him, brushing the snow from his overcoat before hanging it in the drying closet.

Woody checked his patient. She carried a large baby; plenty of time remained. He unpacked and set up the portable delivery table alongside his patient's bed. An hour passed, another, then another. The cervix was now fully dilated; it was time to shift the patient to the delivery table. Woody applied forceps and eased the baby girl through the birth canal. She cried vigorously, and someone in the outer room cheered. A neighbor lady assisted in sponging the baby, whom she then placed next to her mother. Woody had experienced fatigue on many prior deliveries, but this one established a record. He cleaned and repacked his instruments and the delivery table before joining the family for a sandwich and bowl of soup.

Woody needed to return to Canton. The first hints of dawn signaled a new day with other responsibilities that would unfold on the other side of the river. The farmer settled accounts, and the two men remounted the tractor for its second shuttle of the day. They reached the dam without incident. The snowfall had diminished.

"I can't thank you enough, Doc," the farmer said.

Woody bade him goodbye before climbing the stairs to the rim of the dam. He was exhausted and glad that the snow had ended and the wind had slackened. He longed for home and a hot shower. In another hour he would realize both.

Among his many home deliveries, this one, having taken place in the middle of a blizzard that made all travel nearly impossible and exceptionally hazardous, would gain the status of legend.

No accurate count exists of the number of babies delivered in the home by Woody Dodson before he hung up his forceps in 1950. Learning of his plans to cease the obstetrical part of his practice, a devoted patient promised to bake him a cake at each of his birthdays if he would see her through her pregnancy and delivery. This delivery, a boy, would be the final one performed by Woody, and the cakes arrived at each of his birthdays until he died forty-seven years later.

Woodrow Bryan Dodson was born in 1914 in Kirksville, Missouri. His father, Job Theodore, had the distinction of holding two degrees — Doctor of Medicine and Doctor of Osteopathy — and a reputation as an inventor. However, when Woody's parents divorced during his childhood his mother assumed full responsibility for supporting her son and herself. Divorce back then stigmatized a family, and Woody spoke very little about those years to his own children. Further marring his boyhood was an eye injury caused by a BB pellet. Glaucoma had ensued in the left eye, then blindness, until finally the eye was replaced with a prosthesis.

Woody attended the Kirksville Teachers College. After graduation he worked for the local newspaper, keeping its office furnace stoked, until he could earn enough money to pursue his real goal — the study of medicine. When he graduated from the Kirksville College of Osteopathic Medicine in 1939, however, he had no savings; all of his wages from part-time jobs during his academic years had been devoted to paying college expenses. The region still suffered the effects of the Great Depression, and there was no prospect of obtaining a loan from a bank to establish an office.

Undaunted, Woody rented a two-room office in nearby LaGrange, Missouri. He slept each night upon the treatment table until he could save enough money to move into a boarding house. Lunch during his years in LaGrange consisted of two bananas and a glass of milk. Some of his patients could pay fifty cents or a dollar for their care, while others traded vegetables or eggs for his services. For two years Woody struggled with little success to build a practice in LaGrange. He met and courted Mary Jane Berryman, whom he married in 1941. Soon after the wedding, he unhesitatingly accepted an offer to join the practice of an older physician in Canton, Missouri and finally gained a financial toehold.

Canton rests on the banks of the Mississippi River. In the early '40s, the small town featured a single stoplight and had neither a pharmacy nor a hospital. Patients who needed inpatient care traveled seventeen miles by car to Quincy, Illinois. Historic Culver-Stockton College was the pride of the town. Founded in 1853, the College had the distinction of being the first institution of higher learning west of the Mississippi founded expressly to educate both men and women.

Not long after Woody's arrival in Canton, his senior partner died. In the subsequent years of his practice, Woody sometimes worked with an associate. For years he was the only physician who resided within the town, and he attended his office six days each week. On Wednesday afternoons he drove to Quincy to purchase the medications that he dispensed at his office. When the small waiting room at the office reached its capacity, patients waited in their cars and trucks for their turn to see the doctor. Woody made house calls most evenings, Saturday afternoons, and Sundays. He cared for patients of all ages.

Lack of money never precluded care. Office visits cost three dollars for those patients with money. Produce or the performance of chores satisfied the accounts of patients without money.

The pace of practice took a toll. Soon after a fire gutted his office in 1953, Woody suffered a heart attack that would require years of convalescence before he could return to full-time work. While he struggled to regain his health, Mary Jane completed academic work for a teacher's certificate to help support the family. After his recovery, Woody sought to simplify his clinical routine by opening an office first in the enclosed back porch, then in a converted den in the family home. Patients waited their turns in cars parked in the Dodson driveway. Many house calls were replaced by nighttime arrivals of the sick and injured at the backdoor of the Dodson home. Eventually, to ease the burden on his household, it was necessary to convert a neighboring garage into an office, which he would use for the remainder of his working years. Regardless of the location of the office, the telephone rang most nights at all hours.

Woody and Mary Jane had four children, two boys and two girls, who revered their father, and Woody carved time from his clinical duties to spend Saturday afternoons either fishing or hiking through nearby woods with his family. Twice during the childhoods of the older two children the family took brief vacations to Texas and to California. Woody found perfect relaxation in baseball, especially as played by the St. Louis Cardinals. If the broadcast of a Cardinal game conflicted with a social obligation or a meeting, Woody wore an earplug connected to a tiny pocket radio. During the autumn and winter he switched his allegiance to the football and basketball teams of the University of Missouri. In later years he stacked two television sets atop one another so that he could follow different games simultaneously. The children delighted in stringing out their goodnight rituals in Woody's bedroom so that they could watch the televised action over their dad's shoulder. Woody additionally devoted a portion of each evening to Bible study and to the reading of an array of medical journals.

Woody also enjoyed golf. In mid-life he required surgery for a tumor on a nerve in his left arm, and, although his left arm remained weakened after the procedure, he never lost his zest for the game. He derived special pleasure in teaching the game to his two younger children. His son Jeff recalls golf's three basic principles as taught by his father — grip, stance, and follow-through.

Aware of his obligations to Canton as a citizen as well as a physician, Woody devoted time to his Masonic Lodge, the Kiwanis Club, and the Chamber of Commerce. He volunteered time for Cub Scouts and Boy Scouts while his sons were young. Only illness would keep Mary Jane and Woody from Sunday School and services at the First Baptist Church. Guests always joined the family for Sunday dinner. Many of the diners were friends from church; others were people whom Woody and Mary Jane sensed in need of companionship or a morale boost. Patients provided a steady stream of vegetables and homemade breads for the family.

Jeff Dodson had the special privilege of serving as his father's driver on many nocturnal and weekend house calls. He remembers the thrill of entering patients' homes with his dad — patients and their families were profuse in their welcomes and expressions of gratitude. "He was a real twenty-four–seven kind of guy," Jeff recalls. Woody commemorated his driver's graduation from high school by taking him to New York City. While there, Woody obtained a new glass eye.

Brenda Dodson, the eldest of Woody and Mary Jane's children, worked as her father's receptionist and office assistant for several years in the late 1970s. She remembers the layout of the clinic. The waiting room opened into a small area where Woody performed eye examinations and fitted glasses. Another room accommodated a treatment table for osteopathic manipulations. By that time the charge for an office visit had risen to seven dollars plus the cost of medication. Brenda recalls, "People would come in and talk to him and they would feel better. He truly believed that God had called him to be a doctor. And he lived that calling."

Never robust after his heart attack at age thirty-nine, Woody nonetheless practiced until 1989. "My work is done," he said at that point. The years following retirement were especially difficult as Mary Jane slipped progressively into the mental limbo of Alzheimer's disease. Woody voiced his profound disappointment that the projects and pleasures that he had postponed until retirement would never be realized.

"I was just starting to enjoy life," he told Brenda. Mary Jane died in January 1997. "I sure do miss my wife," Woody lamented. Woody's health steadily deteriorated, and he died in Canton in December 1997.

I met Woody once when he came to Chattanooga to visit his son David, an internist and my partner for twenty years. A slender, elegant, white-haired man with a pronounced Midwestern accent, he came to view our big city office one Saturday. I recall his turning to me before his departure to tell me, "You have a really fine clinic here." I wonder in retrospect if he did not think our office with its multiple specialized rooms to be extravagant in the extreme. I suspect that in a typical day he saw more patients than I ever saw in one of my typical days, and he provided care to his people in a fourth of the space that I depended upon.

Especially during the first decade or so of my own practice I encountered many older patients who longed for care by a fabled general practitioner from their past. "Why can't we go back to those days?" they would ask.

Almost all of these individuals had a memory of a physician whom they saw either in an office or during a home visit. That physician had a magical presence, representing comfort, knowledge, and skill precisely attuned to the moment. Scarlet fever or diphtheria or a childhood fracture might be the event precipitating the visit with the physician. Whether in the office or the home, options for evaluation and treatment were limited. My mother recalls her family's physician coming to her home to suture a severe laceration of her tongue when she was six years old. A seesaw had struck her chin, and her teeth had almost severed her tongue. After administering ether to his patient, the doctor expertly repaired the injury. My own memories relate to my great-uncle Ruben O'Neal, whose gentle yet authoritative visits to my bedside during times of illness epitomized professional concern. His presence signaled security.

In those days an injection might be administered or a prescription given for a medication that the pharmacist would concoct. Admission to hospital was reserved for very ill patients. In the eye of memory, at least, the physician seemed to be a savior from dire predicaments, whatever the setting. Paradoxically, the same individuals who now long for the physician of old more often than not expect referral to specialists to address the malfunctioning of each organ system. Most patients who are middle-aged and younger have no memories of these seemingly magical physicians of not so long ago.

Would Woody Dodson today be an anachronism?

Clearly he had a vision of service. Perhaps he acquired this from his physician-father. Woody never considered practice in a large city. He was comfortable among the varied people of the farms and small towns in the Heartland. Like them, he had been raised in the traditions of hard work and neighborliness. A candid photograph of Woody administering immunizations to school children captures a gentle, reassuring smile directed toward the frightened little girl who is about to be stuck. She is not a number but someone whose care Woody takes very seriously. Probably none of his patients would have noticed if Woody had been lax in keeping his medical knowledge current, but as a matter of intellectual pride he studied most nights. He did not have the luxury of teleconferences or postgraduate seminars, but he developed and adhered to his own, personal standard of excellence: no patient would suffer because he was ill-informed. His medical career defines commitment and compassion.

Woody's career-long commitment to his work took multiple tolls. Exhaustion contributed to a heart attack. A variety of projects that he had postponed for retirement were precluded by Mary Jane's, and then his own, failed health. At various times his marital relationship suffered from the seemingly unending clinical demands. The Great Depression mandated habits of intense, unrelieved work from which many men and women who grew into maturity during those years could never relinquish. Having witnessed financial ruin among their friends and relatives, they never felt really secure.

Because he had come from a broken home, Woody cherished his role as father. Many times, however, his four children could catch little more than glimpses of their father. There was no answering service to manage the torrent of telephone calls and, often, no other physician to whom Woody might sign out. Brenda reflects, "We children paid the price." When patients thanked Woody for his devotion to their well-being, they should have thanked his family as well. The sacrifices of his clinical service to his community involved all six members of the family in different ways.

Woody Dodson's career has many parallels in family physicians of the twentieth century. Most of these careers are recalled only within the community in which the physician worked, but one such career is a poignant exception. In 1967 John Berger's *A Fortunate Man* was published, an account of an English general practitioner, John Sassall, who served the residents of a poor rural area. Berger spent a number of days with the doctor as he conducted his clinic and made house calls to his far-flung patients. Photographer Jean Mohr captured moving images of the physician at work.

Sassall treated children and adults, and he offered close bedside support to his dying patients. He spoke quite candidly to Berger of his love for his work but also of the fatigue and depression which that work generated. Like Woody Dodson, John Sassall served as a domestic medical missionary. *A Fortunate Man* has been rightly extolled for its portrayal of a selfless, dedicated physician.

In 2001 an essay in *The Lancet* reported that Dr. Sassall had died by his own hand several years earlier. When the author, J.S. Huntley, visited the town in which Sassall had practiced, he found that few of its residents remembered or had knowledge of him. Huntley located the tombstone of only the doctor's wife in the village churchyard and presumed that suicide had precluded Dr. Sassall's burial in sacred ground. The gloomy prospect arises that the citizens of the area exhausted Dr. Sassall and simply forgot him once he could no longer be of immediate service.

Four years after Woody Dodson's death, his daughter Anne, who teaches in the Canton schools, frequently encounters former patients of her father. They speak of his devotion to them, of special assistance that he rendered when tragedy struck a family, of the vigil that he maintained at the bedside of a dying grandmother. For a generation, at least, the memory of Woody seems secure in the hearts of those he tended.

Another memorial to Woody persists in the career of his son David, an internist in Chattanooga whose practice, though based in the hospital of a big city, brings to the bedside of his patients the compassion and commitment of a man who once crossed a dam in a snowstorm to deliver a baby.

In a recent alumni publication I read of a two-year initiative to rework the undergraduate medical curriculum at the Johns Hopkins University School of Medicine. The challenge of incorporating the advances of genomic medicine and the boundless other technologic advances drove the conversation among distinguished academicians. In an already packed curriculum, additional time had to be carved out for revolutionary concepts in human biology. The questions were twofold: what course work would be added and what would be dropped.

I hope that in all such technologically sophisticated institutions someone will regularly hold up for study and for veneration the careers of quietly great physicians such as Woodrow Dodson and John Sassall. Quite obviously, these physicians define devotion to patients. Their careers also raise important issues of boundaries. The necessarily demanding work of clinical medicine must be balanced and humanized by time spent with family and friends and by time for reflection outside the medical sphere.

Many physicians in my generation entered medicine because we admired the physicians who took care of us when we were sick or injured, but our role models are now gone. When our generation passes from the scene there will few links to a time of intense, personal commitment by medical doctors to the welfare of their patients, no matter the setting, the hour, or the economics.

On behalf of all his patients, I thank Woodrow Dodson, Doctor of Osteopathy.

SOURCES AND ACKNOWLEDGMENTS

Woody and Mary Jane's children, Brenda, David, Jeffrey, and Anne, granted interviews and patiently answered many questions. *A Fortunate Man* (1967) by John Berger, photographs by Jean Mohr, is available in paperback. J.S. Huntley honors Dr. Sassall in a fine essay, "In Search of *A Fortunate Man*," in *The Lancet* (2001;357:546–49).

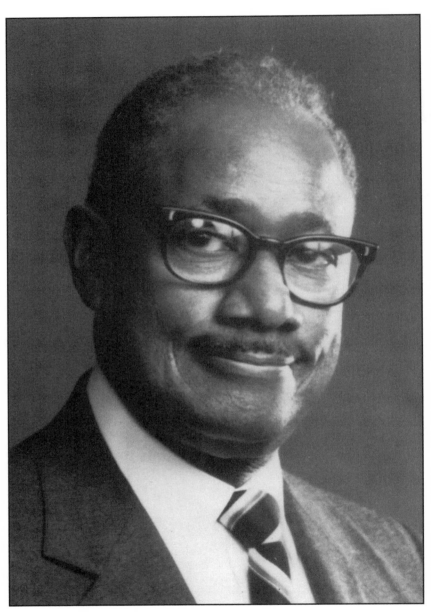

Dr. Lonnie Boaz Jr.

THE JANITOR IN THE EYE CLINIC; OR, BROOMS, MOPS, AND OPHTHALMOSCOPES: LONNIE BOAZ JR.

—◦◦◦—

The operator paged me. "Doctor Boaz is on the phone. He says it's urgent."

When Lonnie Boaz said "urgent" he meant it. I answered at once.

"Clif, I have a man in my office, and I think he has tuberculosis in his neck. I'd like to send him over."

Lonnie informed me that the patient, a retired janitor, had come to his office stating that his right shoulder ached with a dull pain that had gradually worsened over the past month and now prevented sleep. The man could not find a comfortable position in which to rest. After examining him, Lonnie had obtained an X-ray of his neck, which showed partial destruction of two of seven cervical vertebrae.

Because it would be necessary to conduct additional tests, I agreed to meet the patient in the emergency room of Erlanger Hospital. He arrived within the hour. His third and fourth cervical vertebrae appeared so moth-eaten in the X-rays that I feared collapse and spinal cord injury. Detailed study during the next few days confirmed that tuberculosis was indeed the culprit. A long interval in a neck brace, months of anti-tuberculosis medication, and surgery to reconstruct the damaged vertebral bodies restored the man to active health, and he went on to live into his early eighties.

"Lonnie, how on earth did you know that was tuberculosis?" I enquired after biopsies and cultures had confirmed the diagnosis.

Lonnie explained to me that he had seen two similar cases during his medical training. He had filed them in the odd part of the brain where all good doctors store their personal clinical experiences. This was but one of many shrewd diagnoses made by my colleague during the overlapping years of our careers.

Both of us were early risers. Many mornings we arrived almost simultaneously at the nursing station on the medical ward. Usually we swapped a joke before commenting upon a story in the morning paper or an issue in hospital politics. Both of us tended toward cynicism, especially during the Nixon and Ford presidential years. With each other, we could articulate our liberal politics without contradiction because no one else was usually around at that hour. Our "lounge" consisted of a counter upon which we could lean while having the morning's second cup of coffee. If we had seen a clinical oddity since our last meeting, we would describe it. I think we both relished our brief daily meeting and arranged our rounds to ensure the continuation of our morning ritual.

Our other meetings occurred at a large Home Depot. Coincidence accounted for these encounters over a ten-year period, always on Wednesday afternoons when we would both take a half-day away from office routines. Lonnie was a man of projects. Once he purchased, after much study and extensive questioning of a clerk, great lengths of irrigation tubing for his lawn and garden. The tubing remained in his garage, awaiting the right moment for installation. Lonnie's wife, Aurellia, contended that he had purchased enough tubing to irrigate large tracts in the Middle East. My purchases were smaller, usually some outdoor gadget that I felt that I had to have and that typically gathered dust in my garage, awaiting some special alignment of the planets that would signal the moment of their use.

Besides planning household projects, Lonnie loved boating on a nearby TVA-lake. I dubbed him "Commodore" after spending a Sunday afternoon touring the lake with him. Afloat, he was a study in serenity, a sharp contrast to his high-energy demeanor in the hospital. That Sunday we made stops at several inlets so he could visit with his boating buddies.

"He could relax just looking at a cup of water," Aurellia later commented.

Our friendship matured over eighteen years, he a black man of the South, and I a white man of the South. As the months and years went on, we expanded the range of our deliberations. Chattanooga continued to struggle with the legacies of segregation during much of that time. Lawsuits and harsh rhetoric periodically dominated front pages. Lonnie and I solved most of these issues in our daily two-man conclaves. Fortunately, the city had calm reformers in both the black and white communities who would eventually transform smoldering rage into faltering steps toward racial integration.

Hattie Boaz gave birth to Lonnie R. Boaz Jr. in 1929 in Hampton, Virginia. She and her husband, Lonnie Sr., then moved to Huntsville, Alabama where the latter joined the faculty of Alabama Agricultural and Mechanical College as an instructor in tailoring. The college had opened its doors in 1875 as Huntsville Normal School to provide vocational training for black Alabamans. Its first president had been a slave. Famed musician W.C. Handy once served as the school's band director. The college prepared its students for work in various trades or for positions as Pullman car porters.

In 1931, Lonnie's father drove with friends to an out-of-town football game. Somehow their car collided with a vehicle occupied by several white men. When additional white men arrived on the scene, a fight ensued. Lonnie Sr. died from injuries sustained in that fight. One week later, Hattie Boaz gave birth to a second son.

Hattie struggled to stabilize her suddenly diminished yet newly enlarged family. While she studied to qualify for a teaching certificate, Lonnie Jr. and his brother lived for a year with relatives in New York City where Lonnie completed first grade. The brothers next moved to Chattanooga to spend a year in the home of their paternal grandmother. A precocious Lonnie skipped second grade and completed third grade at Orchard Knob Elementary School, and the happiness of that year would influence later choices in his life.

Finally, Hattie reunited her family in Hampton, where she taught in an elementary school. Lonnie's part-time and summer jobs helped support the family. After graduation from high school, he worked for a year in home construction to save money for tuition at Hampton Institute, at which he enrolled in 1944 to study business. Military service called in 1945. Trained as a medic, Lonnie served in the eye clinic at Fitzsimmons Army Hospital in Denver. He learned refraction as well as diagnosis and treatment of minor eye disorders. This experience would cast the die for Lonnie's subsequent pursuit of a career in medicine.

After he was honorably discharged from the Army in 1946, Lonnie returned to the Hampton Institute, this time to major in chemistry and biology. Summer and after-class work as a house painter provided the cash for books and tuition. A second job as a janitor took Lonnie to the military hospital at Langley Air Force Base. When the medical officers learned of Lonnie's background in ophthalmology, they arranged for him to split his time between the eye clinic and his janitorial duties.

Although financial stresses once again forced a one-year pause in college, in 1949 Lonnie married Aurellia Mitchell, whom he had first met in a botany class. While she worked as a research mathematician at Langley, Lonnie returned to Hampton, completing his bachelor's degree in 1951. He entered medical school at Howard University, and in 1955 the janitor who did eye work received his Doctor of Medicine degree. Internship in Winston Salem preceded his move to Chattanooga where he would spend his career. In time, two sons and a daughter were born to complete his family.

When Lonnie moved to Chattanooga in 1956, he could admit his patients only to Carver Memorial Hospital on the city's west side. The board of trust for all-white Erlanger Hospital managed all-black Carver as if it were a missionary hospital in a foreign country. Should a patient at Carver need blood, his nurse would dispatch a janitor by taxi to retrieve units of blood from the laboratory at Erlanger Hospital.

When Carver Hospital fell to a wrecking ball in 1959, Erlanger Hospital rushed to complete a west wing for black physicians and their patients. Years would pass before the chasm of segregation could be bridged between the two wings of the "unified" hospital. Meanwhile, Lonnie gained membership on the staffs of two other hospitals within the city.

I had known segregated hospitals from my medical school experience in Baltimore where the Johns Hopkins Hospital segregated the races with separate floors for black and white patients. I did not see one black student, house officer, or faculty member in that hospital during my three-year stay from 1961 to 1964. At Vanderbilt Hospital in Nashville where I served my internship in medicine, black and white patients were housed on the same floor but never shared rooms. I did not know enough or feel enough at the time to question this practice.

It was quite inadvertently that I had integrated a ward in Vanderbilt Hospital late one evening. A black bartender, whom I had admitted to the teaching service, had begun to vomit large amounts of blood, and his blood pressure fell. Our ward had a two-bed special care unit, a primordial intensive care unit, in which severely ill patients could receive closer monitoring and nursing care than was available on the rest of the floor. Knowing there was a vacancy, I enlisted an orderly to help me push the bed bearing my bleeding patient into the special-care room. His roommate was a white man, also my patient, who suffered from severe rheumatoid arthritis and heart failure.

The head nurse exploded, "You can't do that!" and told me I would be reported. If I was reported, however, nothing ever came of it. Both of my patients improved. Neither objected to the presence of the other. The families of each, though initially wary of one another, made efforts at conversation. On the medical service of Vanderbilt Hospital segregation slowly faded away.

Unlike Erlanger Hospital, Chattanooga's city-county medical society would need additional years before accepting the membership application of Lonnie Boaz and other black physicians in 1964. Prior to that decision Lonnie had served for a decade as president of the Mountain City Medical Society, which black physicians had organized. Informal racial barriers persisted in the hospital and in the city-county medical society for long after this time. Lonnie refused for years to enter the physicians' lounge of Erlanger Hospital because he felt unwelcome there.

"I went once and heard them talking about me behind my back. I didn't need that."

Decades later Erlanger Hospital, the city of Chattanooga, and much of the South still continue the struggle toward racial harmony. In August 2003 I listened to a conversation that illustrates the uphill nature of that struggle. My wife and I had taken three of our grandchildren to the Tennessee Valley Railroad Museum where we boarded a restored passenger train which took us along a route that included a Civil War era tunnel beneath Missionary Ridge, the site of a bloody Union victory in 1863. An on-board guide and conductor pointed out various historic sites and briefly mentioned the battle between Union and Confederate armies. A church group from Alabama shared our coach. After we passed through the tunnel, the elderly leader of the group loudly intoned that if he had been alive in 1863, "I would have killed me a bunch of those Yankees. We would never have given up, and things wouldn't be in the mess they are today." No one chuckled. A fellow parishioner replied, "Amen, brother." The rest of us contemplated our shoes.

Lonnie delivered babies at Carver Hospital, set fractures, and treated medical problems of adults and children in his office at 1620 South Market Street. He had selected that location because of its ease of access to city bus service. House calls enlivened many of his evenings. Somehow Lonnie found extra hours to serve on boards and committees of the YMCA, the Georgia-Tennessee Regional Health Commission, Fairview Presbyterian Church, and the Metropolitan Council for Community Services. In 1972 he assumed the chairmanship of the family practice section of Erlanger Hospital. In 1987 he accepted the mayor's appointment to that hospital's board of trustees.

Late in the evening of January 30, 1990, I received another call from a Dr. Boaz, but this time the caller was Dr. Valerie Boaz, Lonnie's daughter. Her father had collapsed, she told me. An ambulance had been summoned. Could I meet them at the Erlanger emergency room.

I arrived moments before the ambulance. Lonnie was deeply comatose. My quick examination suggested that he had bled into his brain. A CT scan confirmed a large amount of blood in the posterior aspect of his brain, and already blood had torn through much of his central nervous system. A neurologist whom I telephoned joined me at the view boxes in the radiology department. From a technical standpoint, much of the accumulated blood could be removed by a neurosurgical procedure. But what kind of life would remain for Lonnie? The neurologist concluded that his life could possibly be preserved; however, he would have substantial disabilities. He might never regain consciousness, spending the rest of his days in a "locked-in" state. He might awaken but not be able to speak or care for himself. We repeated our examination of Lonnie. Every sign indicated severe damage to his brain.

Lonnie did not have a "living will," but at various times in our meetings during morning rounds, Lonnie and I had exchanged our deepest held views on life, death, and illness. Neither of us wanted to live if we could not think, if we could not express and enjoy the love of our families.

I met Aurellia and the children — businessman Andre, Dr. Valerie, and Dr. Lonnie III — in one of the so-called "family" rooms that all hospitals maintain for such times of sadness and difficult decisions. I reviewed the results of the studies that had been quickly completed. We considered the man, his relish for life, his love of medicine, and the grim outlook for recapturing that life. We prayed. Unanimously, Lonnie's family elected comfort care for their patriarch. Meanwhile, the waiting room of the emergency department had filled with friends, patients, and community leaders who had learned of Lonnie's calamity. They came together to mourn, to express sympathy to Lonnie's family, and to comfort each other.

In a quiet, private room in Erlanger Hospital, the hospital that he had helped to integrate through his gentle leadership, Lonnie Boaz — physician, husband, father, civic leader and reformer, one-time painter, janitor, and medic, son of a victim of a hate crime, life member of the National Association for the Advancement of Colored People — died the following morning.

I become angry at times. I harbor grudges and have to work to prevent such emotions from corroding my days. On several occasions when I was nursing a grievance, I asked Lonnie how he remained calm. I needed to know how he maintained equanimity in the face of the numerous offenses and intimidations of racism. Why had he not opted to settle in a northern or midwestern city where racial battles had been settled? Were there not easier options for an aspiring black physician? How did he avoid throwing up his hands in dismay or disgust?

"I am comfortable here," he responded.

A year as a third grader at Orchard Knob Elementary School and in the home of his grandmother provided a sense of home unlike any other in Lonnie's educational odyssey. Lonnie had felt that he could make a difference in this community even if years would be needed to do so. He was well versed in patience and determination.

Orchard Knob School derives its name from the adjacent site of a skirmish of the Civil War battles of Chattanooga. Confederate forces had fortified the hundred-foot-tall hill with breastworks and trenches. Orchard Knob was the strongpoint of a lengthy Confederate line behind which lay Missionary Ridge, occupied by powerful Confederate forces. Union forces had slowly increased their strength during months of encirclement in Chattanooga. On November 23, 1863 Union forces massed a mile to the east of Orchard Knob. They drilled before launching an attack in early afternoon. During the first half-mile of their charge, Union forces encountered no opposition. Then, rebel riflemen on Orchard Knob and Confederate artillery atop Missionary Ridge opened fire. Hand-to-hand combat followed as Union forces fought over the breastworks and up the hill. By mid-afternoon the American flag flew over Orchard Knob. Both sides suffered heavy losses — Confederate soldiers from Alabama, Union fighters from Illinois and Ohio. Orchard Knob became headquarters for General Grant as he directed the subsequent victorious assault upon Missionary Ridge.

Granite monuments, artillery pieces, and metal plaques atop Orchard Knob commemorate those who died, were wounded, or simply disappeared in the fighting on the hillside. At issue was whether slavery would be permitted within the United States. Although a Union victory ensured abolition of slavery and emancipation of slaves, racial prejudice continues to haunt the states of the former Confederacy. A different kind of monument, invisible, erected in the hearts of his family and admirers, memorializes a quieter, more sustained, struggle, that of Lonnie Boaz to make his city a kinder place for all God's children.

SOURCES AND ACKNOWLEDGMENTS

I am grateful to Aurellia Boaz and her children who shared with me their memories of Lonnie Boaz. For information on the Battle of Orchard Knob and other aspects of the larger Civil War battles in and around Chattanooga, I depended upon Peter Cozzens', *The Shipwreck of Their Hopes: The Battles for Chattanooga* (University of Illinois Press, Urbana and Chicago, 1994).

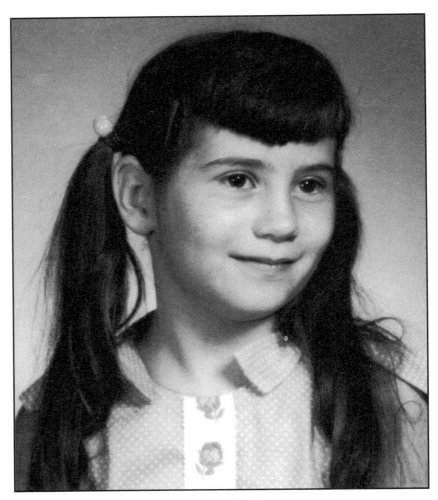

Paulette McGill

CHYLOMICRONS
AND HOLSTEINS:
PAULETTE McGILL

———⁓∾⁓———

She died ten years ago at thirty-two years of age. Perhaps her premature death had been inevitable from the time of conception, for she had both juvenile diabetes and a severe inherited disorder of fat metabolism. Even in childhood her cholesterol and triglyceride values reached levels seldom seen by experts at university centers. Laboratory technicians who processed samples of her blood over the years were repeatedly astounded by the cream-of-tomato-soup appearance of her blood. When a tube of her blood sat undisturbed for an hour, the fluid above the red cells assumed the appearance of thick dairy cream. A thin layer of fat — composed of chylomicrons or microscopic clusters of fatty acids — congealed above this. Within her circulation high levels of cholesterol produced premature atherosclerosis, while chylomicrons repeatedly formed microscopic plugs in her smallest blood vessels, precipitating painful injury to various tissues of her body. Most children with this particular disorder of fat metabolism die in infancy. Her plight showed up in at least one review article in a medical journal. The consulting experts advised a variety of therapies, all of which failed.

Her chart is three and a half inches thick and rests in a locked file. I cannot surrender it to microfilming. I suspect that it serves the role of a memorial to a brave little girl who grew into womanhood during the twenty years in which I served as her primary care physician. The worn cover is pink with various colored tabs along one border to facilitate filing. My nurse had written "Deceased 9-5-93" upon its front cover.

I became Paulette's physician in 1972 because of a lecture that I presented soon after moving to Chattanooga to launch my practice. My talk dealt with inherited abnormalities of blood fats — cholesterol and triglycerides. In reviewing my notes from that talk, which I had given during medical grand rounds at Erlanger Hospital, I saw that I had described the disorder from which Paulette suffered as Type V hyperlipoproteinemia and wondered whether our use of Roman numerals is supposed to give extra gravity to a classification or an event. There was at that time no treatment.

A distinguished local pediatrician, Pope Holliday, attended my talk and afterwards sought my opinion on a twelve-year-old girl, Paulette McGill, who had been his patient for several years. She suffered from brittle diabetes and recurrent bouts of severe abdominal pain attributed to thick, fat-laden blood. I felt honored by such a request from one of the pillars of my city's medical community, although I could not then anticipate all of the lessons, blessings, and heartaches I would experience during my twenty years of association with "our mutual patient," as Dr. Holliday referred to her.

Soon after our curbside consultation, Dr. Holliday asked that I evaluate Paulette. She had been admitted to the children's hospital with chest pain and elevation of her blood glucose. Studies failed to uncover a cause for her chest pain. Her blood sugars responded to insulin and intravenous fluids. The hospital laboratory reported fasting cholesterol levels of one thousand and triglyceride levels of eight thousand. Dr. Holliday asked if I would accept responsibility for Paulette's continuing medical care.

Usually, I do not assume the care of patients until they are fifteen or older. Sometimes boys and girls who mature early want to graduate from the waiting rooms of pediatricians to the offices of internists, or "doctors for grown-ups" as one teenaged patient stated it. For whatever reason, Paulette determined that my office would be her medical home. Often, during our long acquaintance, she enquired of Dr. Holliday's health and asked that I relay to him her greetings. Similarly, whenever I would encounter Dr. Holliday he would enquire of

Paulette's well-being and would ask that I convey to her his best wishes. Like most pediatricians whom I have known over the years, Pope Holliday maintained an active file in his heart for every patient he had treated. This master pediatrician invested a little bit of his soul in each of his patients.

Paulette never grew beyond the fifty-nine-inch height that my nurse recorded at the time of her first visit to our office. Her appearance was that of perpetual youth.

From the time of Paulette's first visit to my office, she insisted upon being evaluated in private. Her mother, who served as her chauffeur until Paulette reached driving age, waited patiently until Paulette signaled my nurse and me that her mother could join us. This reflected no animosity. Paulette aspired early to be an independent and a responsible director of her own medical care. She asked questions, made notes, and reviewed her plans for coming weeks.

Few patients could claim the level of meticulous care that Paulette devoted to controlling her diabetes. She maintained detailed records of her blood glucose levels and was expert in gauging how much insulin she might need in a variety of circumstances. Despite her best efforts, however, Paulette, from her late teen years onward, suffered repeated episodes of retinal bleeding that required many laser treatments. When faced with a sudden change in vision, she never evinced fear or exasperation. Her concerns dealt with how soon she could resume her normal activities. Paulette announced quite early in our association that she had two special missions in life — to teach kindergarten and to perform musically. Her desire for a teaching career grew from her work as a volunteer in vacation Bible school in the South Rossville Baptist Church of Rossville, Georgia. She could not recall when her love of music began. She studied piano and had taught herself to play the organ, violin, and flute.

At the end of the technical part of a visit when we would review blood sugars, discuss diet, and look at patterns of any recent insulin reactions, Paulette routinely steered the conversation toward more personal issues. She welcomed questions about her work in school, her favorite subjects, a book she might be reading for a formal report. If a recent school test had not gone well, she reported where her study had been inadequate or off target.

"Exactly what does a kindergarten teacher do, Paulette?" I asked one day as she approached graduation from high school.

"They do everything. They teach about letters, colors, and music. They teach about love."

The topic of love came up repeatedly in her conversations. An only child, she felt profoundly cherished by her parents, James and Pauline. Repeatedly, she stated how blessed she was to be a part of that particular family. The idea that children could be unloved or, worse still, could ever experience abuse at the hands of a parent or any adult caused her pain. Should a Chattanooga newspaper or television station report an incident of child abuse, Paulette would ask "why" and "what can we do" at the time of her next visit.

Paulette always seemed to believe that my nurse and I needed to have our spirits boosted. She greeted us warmly on each visit, shaking our hands. She dressed cheerfully, always wearing a skirt and, depending upon the season, a brightly colored vest or blouse. One day, while still in high school, she appeared in black and white. Irregular, black patches adorned her white skirt. Smaller, ovoid patches of black had been inked onto her white socks and canvas sneakers. She was quick to tell us that this was her Holstein attire.

"I thought it would give you a laugh," she said to us.

Paulette completed all of her schooling at Tennessee Temple, an independent Baptist school system in Chattanooga. With the approach of graduation from high school in 1980 she grew impatient to begin collegiate work. She had already mapped out which classes she would take and in what sequence once she matriculated at Tennessee Temple University. She had already selected elementary education as her academic major. Perhaps her impatience derived from a sense that her health might become a limiting issue in her plans. Occasional bouts of abdominal pain, increasingly fragile diabetes, and episodes of retinal bleeding slowed but never stopped her academic progress. Whenever she lost time because of hospitalization, she quickly doubled her pace of study to avoid falling behind.

Practice teaching reaffirmed for Paulette that she was placed in this life expressly to teach. Her excitement became almost palpable as she discussed lesson plans and her interactions with students. Paulette seemed truly amazed that preschoolers called her "Miss McGill."

On graduation day from college I delivered a small gift to Paulette at her home. "I did it, Dr. Cleaveland, I did it!" She bounced with excitement. Her tears flowed freely. She gave me the tassel from her graduation cap, which today hangs on my framed medical degree.

Acquiring a job proved a problem for the new graduate. Paulette wanted to teach in a Christian school, but because of her diabetic history several potential employers turned her away. Some employers may have worried that diabetes would lead to excessive absenteeism on her part. Her illness would drive health insurance premiums upward for small, self-insured schools. A couple of jobs were available if she would sign a one-year waiver for any health care related to diabetes, but, finally, a principal at an independent school in her home community offered a contract to her to teach kindergarten with no strings attached, and her career was off and running.

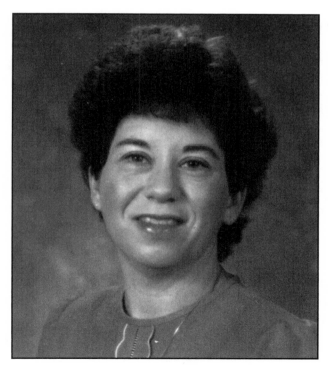

Paulette McGill as the teacher she dreamed of becoming.

In December of that first year Paulette lost vision in her right eye. An inflammation of unknown cause necessitated a stay in the hospital and extensive outpatient follow-up with retinal specialists. Perhaps fatty globules in the tiniest of retinal arteries initiated the process.

"When can I go back to work?" This would be her repeated question during the coming years. She lived to teach.

Paulette's best efforts to control her diabetes faltered as she required larger and larger doses of insulin. She had to cope with increasingly frequent episodes of abdominal pain, and her blood fat levels soared despite every available medication and the best efforts of consultants in nearby university medical centers. Sometimes her abdominal pain derived from pancreatitis, the presumption being that microscopic fat droplets in her blood blocked the smallest blood vessels in her pancreas causing severe injury to the cells of that vital gland. Sometimes the process attacked the walls of her intestine or her kidneys. Whatever the site of injury, she experienced pain that in its intensity rivaled acute appendicitis.

Many days Paulette taught in constant discomfort. She realized the implications for her career should she lose too many days to illness. When she had to yield to pain and seek further help, she would simply say, "Please help me." She never cried out. She seldom requested medication for pain either in the office or in the hospital. When hospitalized, she dealt with pain by closing her eyes and concentrating upon pieces of music. At times of particularly intense pain she hummed hymns. She appeared severely pale at such times. Never did she articulate the question, "Why me?" I, on the other hand, often thought "Why Paulette? Why anyone, for that matter?"

Repeatedly, I have heard religious counselors tell someone who is suffering that "The Lord never puts upon us more than we can bear." Paulette and I discussed this aphorism once after she had heard it used at a funeral. She could not imagine a loving God ever inflicting an illness such as hers upon anyone. We agreed that our bodies suffered various illnesses and injuries because we were biological entities, subject to innumerable malfunctions in the complex machinery of our bodies. We shared a view that God infused our frail bodies with strength and love that was independent of our biological nature.

She lost her job — too many days absent — and no one else would hire her. She tried substitute teaching. She submitted one resume after another, answered advertisements, consulted placement agencies. Finally, an independent school in another city took a chance on her. She loved the school, the children, and her colleagues on the faculty and staff.

"How are things going?" was my standard inquiry about her recent weeks at work.

"They are going great!"

"How are the kids?"

"They are wonderful!"

Paulette took special delight in reading to her students, usually stories with a Biblical theme but also *Winnie the Pooh* and *Charlotte's Web*. If her class behaved well, she rewarded them with music from her flute. I have never seen a happier, more contented person in any job.

Eventually, though, the attacks of abdominal pain intensified and became more frequent. Despite a particularly severe episode in the autumn of 1992, Paulette felt that she had to return to work earlier than desirable for fear that she would lose her position. I sought renewed advice from experts in fatty disorders. No new therapy had been devised.

She wrote on November 2 to report her blood sugars:

Hi, Dr. Cleaveland,

My blood sugars have been high since I've had a strep throat. I'm feeling better now, but my energy is slow in returning. There are all sorts of viruses and colds already going through my classroom. I have a different group of children out each week — I suppose we'll all survive! I'm anxious for a vacation. It won't be long until it's time to visit you — see you soon!

Love,

Paulette

Paulette sent postcards and notes when away from the city. She favored folded notes that depicted smiling mice, puppies, or rabbits on the front page. She especially liked pictures of Dalmatians, spotted like her Holstein outfit. A smiling face accompanied the salutation of each note. Once she traveled to Hawaii — "My extravagant vacation," she called it. Postcards documented the sights and the status of her blood sugar levels.

Christmas vacation brought Paulette unrelenting abdominal pain and a new problem. Circulation to the toes of her right foot had failed. Vascular studies showed blockage of the smallest arteries in her lower legs and feet. Surgical treatment was not feasible. Amputation of her right foot would soon be necessary, but Paulette wanted to delay this as long as possible. The toes turned black, and a podiatrist worked tirelessly to limit the damage. Reluctantly, Paulette applied for long-term disability through the Social Security Administration. Twice her claim was denied.

She mourned the forced absence from her students, but she continued to find peace and happiness in playing piano and organ at services and celebrations in her home church.

Three days after providing piano accompaniment for a Wednesday night prayer service, Paulette phoned shortly before midnight.

"Dr. Cleaveland, this is Paulette. I'm scared. My chest hurts so badly."

I urged transport to the hospital by ambulance, but Paulette chose a more comforting ride in her father's car.

We reached the hospital's emergency room at the same time. She smiled from a gurney, gave a weak wave, and died. We were not able to revive her.

In August 2003 my wife and I paid a visit to Pauline McGill to request permission to write about her daughter and found that Paulette's father had died earlier in the year.

"James never got over her death. We loved her so much," her mother told us.

Pauline showed me photographs of a baby, a six-year-old girl, a high school student, a college graduate. Paulette's countenance never changed. Each face showed the hint of a smile and conveyed the sense that the subject had a secret. I think that secret was a deep awareness of what love of life and of the children of this life are all about. Pauline spoke of the occasional visits of her daughter's closest friends and their reminiscences of shared times in the neighborhood or school or church. As I hold her medical file, I think of my two decades of friendship in a medical setting.

I asked her once which hymn was her favorite. She paused for a moment, stated a love for many traditional hymns, then named "God of Grace and God of Glory."

This is its first stanza:

God of Grace and God of Glory,
On Thy people pour Thy power.
Crown Thine ancient church's story,
Bring her bud to glorious flower.
Grant us wisdom, grant us courage,
For the facing of this hour,
For the facing of this hour.

"Grace, wisdom, courage . . . for the facing of this hour."

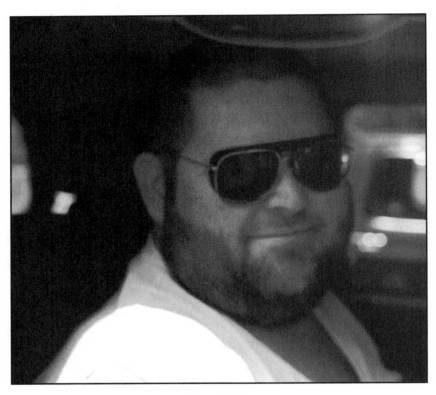

Barry Walker

DIESEL HEARSE:
BARRY WALKER

—◈—

Parked alongside the funeral home, the large Freightliner tractor seemed out of place. A number of other tractors, some with trailers attached, rested further away in the parking lot, at the fringe of all the cars that had transported mourners. This tractor of midnight blue and silver glistened in the morning sunshine. The men without exception paused for a closer look at this diesel marvel before they entered the chapel. Wives or girl-friends waited patiently for them to complete their inspections.

We had come to pay our last respects to Barry Walker. His open coffin rested in a parlor set aside for visitation, and for two days fellow long-distance drivers had taken the several-mile detour from Interstate 75 to say their farewells to their colleague. They joined family, neighbors, friends, fellow church members, and former teachers in a slow, steady procession. Occasionally, one of these visitors placed a note or a small object of remembrance inside the coffin. Each of us paused, perhaps for a moment of prayer, perhaps to call up a memory.

Barry's body was clad in one of his favorite flannel shirts. The artistry of the undertakers had achieved the appearance of peaceful sleep in a man whom we all recalled as bursting with energy. Some mourners wept softly, others smiled. In small clusters men and women exchanged stories. Oral histories begin at such times.

Barry had appeared in my office ten years earlier. Although his diabetes had been diagnosed only two years before our first meeting, the disease had unleashed a relentless and aggressive attack on his body. At a
height of six feet, four inches and a weight of three hundred pounds,
Barry had a formidable presence. A disarmingly gentle and engaging spirit
inhabited his large body. He professed an enduring religious faith that
directed his avoidance of tobacco and alcohol, although he acknowledged
that he was addicted to snacks. During long-distance drives for his truck-
ing firm, he routinely stocked the cab with large cans of potato chips, Little Debbie cakes, and a cooler of soft drinks. Previous physicians had
urged that he adopt a rigorous diet, but he doubted he could maintain
such an unrealistic tactic: any initial resolution he would make wavered
and then collapsed as soon as he drove his rig onto the highway. His
eating exploits assumed the status of legend among fellow drivers. He
promised me that he would try to diet, but he warned that I should not
hold out much hope for success in this venture.

Barry cited a number of reasons that he could not take insulin —
inconvenience, lack of any reproducible schedule, aversion to needles
of any kind. No, insulin was out of the question, he told me. I did convince him to check his blood glucose levels on a portable meter, to
weigh himself whenever he had an opportunity, and to take the pills
for his diabetes on a regular schedule.

Neither then nor at subsequent visits to the office could I ever
muster criticism of Barry and his cavalier approach to his illness. He
had a charisma that would have ensured success in any political contest
that he might have chosen to enter. In the waiting room he struck up
conversations with anyone seated around him. Each member of the
staff who encountered him felt that she had been given entry to his
friendship. His penetrating gaze and firm handshake immediately
conferred comfort and trust upon whomever he greeted. He was not
a manipulator. He did not take any contact lightly or casually. He delighted in banter and swapped stories. In the waiting room he routinely
became the center of a conversational circle that would form around
him.

Barry cited his driving schedule as the cause of missed appoint-
ments. Sometimes his weight dropped a few pounds. Once his weight

even dropped into the mid-two sixties. I suspect that he dieted more rigidly in the days before his infrequent office visits so that his blood glucose levels might fall into a more acceptable range, which they did not.

In 1995, after a two-year absence, he came to see me. His eyes showed early diabetic changes. Protein appeared for the first time in his urine samples. Diabetes had slowly eroded his health. I restated the case for tight control of his diabetes — diet, insulin, and medication to slow the damage to his circulation — but these were boundaries that he could not accept. As engaging as ever, he told me that he would take care of his health in his own way.

Some physicians dismiss patients from their practice if they do not adhere to recommended treatment plans or correct harmful habits. Many more of us try to maintain a patient-doctor relationship even when our advice seems to be discounted. Perhaps we believe that we will eventually prevail in our advocacy for changed life-styles. More likely, we see within our patients certain characteristics that we also share and hence cannot honestly condemn. I never gave up the quest to convince Barry to care for his diabetes. Would it have made a differ-ence in the coming collapse of his health? I do not know. Sometimes diabetes, and most other illnesses as well, behave in totally unpre-dictable fashions. Sometimes the most carefully followed treatment plan will not slow a disease at all. Sometimes a patient may ignore an illness and for many years seem none the worse. These instances force humility upon us. Our word is not law. It is to be considered advice in the light of an uncertain science that races ahead of us.

Barry found love and married. For a time he tightened his diet, monitored his levels of blood sugar, even consented to try insulin therapy. An innately happy man became joyous. Within months, however, his health rapidly deteriorated. Retinal hemorrhages became larger and more numerous and weakened his vision. His kidneys failed. Sensing that he would soon be disabled, Barry ended his marriage. He did not want to be a burden to his wife or to anyone else.

Progressive bleeding in both eyes blinded Barry in 1999. Eye sur-geons removed the vitreous gel from both his eyes. This procedure and numerous laser treatments restored sufficient vision for Barry to read larger print and to drive his pickup truck. No longer qualified to drive commercially, however, Barry worked on a loading dock, placing cargo inside the highway behemoths that he had loved to pilot. He hoped that he would eventually be able to return to the highways, but even his job loading freight had to be surrendered when he suffered further loss of kidney function.

Dialysis ensued, three times weekly. Nurses and technicians at the dialysis center reported that Barry entertained and engaged everyone with whom he came in contact. He listened, told stories, and worked hard to lift the spirits of any fellow patient who seemed downcast. Barry called the dialysis team his "kidney friends." Known for many practical jokes, Barry acknowledged that final mastery in the joke department belonged to his renal team:

One July afternoon while on dialysis, Barry had fallen into a deep sleep. The dialysis staff quickly brought from storage all of their Christmas decorations and attire. Barry awoke in a room replete with Yuletide trappings. "Jingle Bells" played in the background. For a moment, Barry seemed puzzled. He checked the date on his digital watch. "You guys got me this time. But watch out," he warned his friends.

Early in 2001 the circulation in Barry's left leg failed. X-ray studies showed severe, diffuse narrowing in the leg's arteries, but surgery was out of the question. Infection developed in an ulcer on the leg and rapidly advanced upward to his knee. Antibiotics could not stem the spread. When faced with the choice of amputation of his leg at mid-thigh or death from progressive infection, Barry found himself in an unimaginable dilemma. Reluctantly, he agreed to surgery.

One month after the operation, Barry, accompanied by his brother, arrived in my office in a wheelchair. He acknowledged that he had been briefly despondent but was now serving notice that he was back at full throttle. He would pursue physical therapy with vigor and dedication. He planned to obtain a prosthetic limb and learn to walk upon it. He brought with him a stout, six-foot-long oak staff. Using this, he pulled himself to his feet and demonstrated to Nurse Jane and me how he could hobble with the support of his staff. He balanced upon his right leg, then shifted his weight onto the staff, which he grasped firmly with both hands, and hopped forward. Although the process was tiring, he could slowly cover short distances across a room or along a hallway. Several visits later, Barry handed me the staff. He wished me to place it in the corner of my examining room. The staff would remain until he could walk independently upon an artificial leg. At that point he would come to the office, claim his staff, and retire it at his home.

When illness forced his retirement, Barry surrendered one home and later modified a mobile home for his needs. He supervised modifications to his pickup truck to allow free movement around his community. His spirits remained at their customary buoyant level. One day at the office he demonstrated precise tight turns going forward and backward in his wheelchair. He boasted that only a trucker could gain such mastery over a wheelchair. Because of persistent pain in his stump, Barry never found an artificial leg that he could comfortably use.

In early 2003 a painful blister appeared on Barry's right heel. Despite antibiotics, aggressive wound care, and the best efforts of physicians and nurses, the infection spread uncontrollably along his right leg. He could no longer travel to my office alone. His brother and sister accompanied him on separate occasions, each expert in the gentle care of Barry's diseased limb. On April 18, Barry reported increased swelling and the worst pain yet in his right thigh. I found the leg swollen, reddened, and tender with multiple large blisters. I could not detect any pulses.

"Doc, I can stand losing one leg. I can't lose the second."

He agreed to hospitalization for high-dose antibiotics in a last ditch effort to eradicate the infection. Three days later, his leg no better, Barry requested that we stop treatment, and he declined surgical consultation. He wished to have two or three more dialyses to give him time to settle some personal business. He assured me that he had no fear whatsoever of death. Before leaving the hospital he requested that I bring Ruzha, my wife, to visit him when he returned. "Doc, I want to see the lady that has had to put up with you."

We visited Barry late on a Saturday afternoon. Despite pain and fever, he sat up in bed, jovial and expansive, the welcoming host to his temporary dwelling. He introduced us to Diedre, a young woman whom Barry described as a special friend. "God realized that Diedre and I have special needs, and He brought us together to look after each other," he told us.

He thanked Ruzha for taking such good care of me so that I could in turn take care of my patients. In an aside to me he reported his plans to go home in a couple of days, and he elicited a pledge from me. "Doc, I want you to speak at my funeral. Promise me that."

I promised. He reiterated his request when I saw him for the final time in the hospital's dialysis unit two days later.

With home health care in place Barry left the hospital on April 21. When he came to the dialysis center two days later, he thanked the staff for their care and attention. He designated the week as Walker Family Week. As part of the celebration he took his mother, sister, brother-in-law, and their four children to the Chattanooga zoo on April 22. Outwardly jovial, he whispered to his sister that he was in terrible pain. He laughed and joked with his nephews and nieces throughout the visit to the zoo. After lunch he spoke privately with his brother-in-law.

"I can't decide when it's time to die. I don't know how much longer I can stand the pain. I don't want any of my friends to think it's suicide when I decide to stop my treatment. Maybe it's God's choice. I hope He will be swift and merciful."

During his Family Week celebration, Barry presented his nieces and nephews with stuffed bears, each with an implanted recording. He addressed each child by the nickname he had assigned to them and followed it with a short rhyme. He closed with the assurance that he would see them in heaven.

The following day at the dialysis clinic the staff found that the shunt in his arm no longer functioned, but he declined a replacement. Instead he invited his caregivers to a party that he had planned for that evening.

Family and friends gathered at Barry's home for snacks, soft drinks, and a special German chocolate cake that he requested for the occasion. Attendees reported that their host was serene and full of stories and memories. After his guests departed, his mother remained for the evening.

Before dawn he awakened her. He described a recurrent dream in which he was on a trip with different destinations. He asked his mother to pray with him for a perfect ending. He ended his prayer with, "Lord, forgive me," and returned to a sleep from which he would not awaken.

Large trucks drive the imagination of males from our first moments outside our cribs. Plastic ducks, stuffed bears, and building blocks will all have their turns, but it is the truck that first captures and then holds our imaginations. Perhaps we can more readily establish a link between the miniature truck in our hands and the various trucks that we spy whenever we are taken in our car-seats on long or short trips. Delivery trucks, fire trucks, army trucks, eighteen-wheelers, pickup trucks — we like them all — small ones that we can cradle in a hand and move back and forth on a table top or large ones that require two hands to lift. It is a fascination that we never lose. A moment came in the life of each of our four sons when it was time to purchase a yellow Tonka truck. They were sturdy, indestructible, and lent themselves to endless hours of play indoors and outside.

★ ★ ★

My Grandfather Reed gave me my prized truck, a dark olive green, metallic Southern Bell telephone truck. White rubber wheels, ladders, telephone poles, and, mounted on a trailer, an augur for drilling the holes for the poles. If I had to pick one toy from memory that was my favorite, hands down, it would be this one. Christopher Robin had his Winnie the Pooh; I had my telephone truck. Years after I forgot or put aside my truck, I found it again in a rummage through the garage at my parents' home. The truck survived a few more years of demanding play by our sons before finally falling apart.

★ ★ ★

At the annual Nashville automobile show, the large tractor units routinely dominated the attention of our sons. Once, three-year-old William vanished at the show. I frantically searched through the crowd until I heard from overhead, "Hi, dad. Look at me." He had found a way to climb high into the cab of a giant Mack tractor. After climbing rungs of a ladder to fetch him, I had no clue how he had managed his entry.

At around the same time, one hundred fifty miles away, three-year-old Barry Walker had disappeared briefly from his home. His mother had frantically searched the neighborhood for him until an unknown lady appeared with Barry in tow. She had come upon him as he followed a garbage truck making its rounds of the neighborhood. From the time Barry could make sentences, he spoke of a desire to drive a dump truck.

At age four Barry was lost again, this time in a large shopping mall. He approached a security guard to report that his mother was lost. The guard asked him if he meant that he was lost, and Barry replied that he knew where he was; it was his mother who had wandered away.

Always much larger than other children of his age, Barry considered himself the protector of his younger sister. When an older boy picked on his third-grade sister, he threatened the assailant with a beating. "If anyone picks upon her, it will be me."

Barry greeted his sister's first date at the door. "This is my sister. You better take good care of her," he commanded.

Because of his size and strength, Barry seemed a natural for football, but in an eighth-grade game he accidentally injured two players on the opposing team. He gave up the sport for fear that he would inadvertently hurt others.

After his graduation from high school, Barry went to work on his first job driving a garbage truck for a nearby community. One early morning, an agitated motorist blocked the truck's progress with his automobile. When Barry dismounted from the cab, the motorist pulled a revolver. Before he could fire Barry knocked him unconscious with a shovel. He then reported the incident to the police who took the still groggy assailant into custody.

Until he secured his first position as a long-distance driver, Barry worked as a bouncer for nightclubs and as a bounty hunter of felons who had jumped bail. Legends of his strength abounded. His happiest years began with his certification as a pilot for massive highway rigs. He prided himself upon keeping his tractor washed and polished so that it sparkled.

I regarded the magnificent tractor that stood alongside the funeral home with special reverence. My patient and friend had considered his long-haul trucks a veritable extension of his body. He had lived for the travel and the fellowship of the open road. This beautifully waxed truck immediately pulled from memory all of my truck-centered experiences — rides in the back of one uncle's pickup, travel in the cab of another uncle's well-drilling rig, explorations of every fire engine I ever encountered. Was this shiny blue and silver truck placed as a special remembrance of Barry?

Closure of the casket signaled Barry's family and friends to make their way to the chapel. Hymns were played. I spoke a eulogy, fulfilling a promise to Barry. Another friend of Barry, a fellow driver who served also as a roving chaplain and counselor at truck stops, read passages from the Bible and reminisced about shared moments on the road. Barry had asked that the chaplain conduct an "altar call" — a chance for anyone who desired to kneel in the front of the chapel to rededicate their lives to the service of God.

The chaplain closed the service with a prayer. The pallbearers marched alongside the casket as it was rolled up the center aisle of the church and then outside. Eight men lifted the casket and gently secured it behind the cab of the blue and silver tractor. Several friends on motorcycles preceded the tractor to the cemetery. After the chaplain read further scriptural verses and gave a benediction, we mingled and talked for a few minutes. I met one of Barry's teachers and his principal from his elementary school days. They were speaking of his rambunctious good humor when, suddenly, a loud blast came from the air horn of the tractor. Barry had instructed his girlfriend to sound the horn fifteen minutes after the benediction so that everyone would be reminded to cease mourning and return to work.

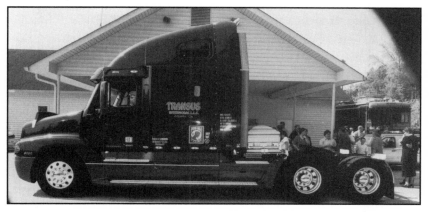

The midnight blue and silver Freightliner that served as hearse for Barry Walker.

Subsequently, I learned that Barry had planned his funeral in detail. He disdained the use of a standard hearse. "I didn't arrive in this life in a Cadillac, and I don't plan to leave it in a Cadillac," he had said. A tractor, similar to the one that he had last driven, would fulfill the role of hearse.

Initially, Barry wanted to schedule his funeral service for seven in the morning. "I always had to wake up early to drive. I want my friends to see what it's like. And I don't want anybody to have to miss work to come." The earlier hour proved impracticable, however, and a ten o'clock service was arranged. At seven that morning a rare earthquake shook our part of the country. At the moment of the tremor, his sister thought, "Barry's in his truck in heaven and he just dumped a load."

★   ★   ★

Years ago American public television imported from Canada a children's program called "The Gentle Giant." The Giant towered over the children and animals of the kingdom. He used his strength to solve simple problems such as rescuing pets or righting a wagon that had turned upon its side. A universal friend, he was welcomed by children and their parents whenever he appeared. Chaos and fear ceased with the arrival of the Gentle Giant. Barry Walker brought the same comfort into the lives of family, friends, care-givers, and even casual acquaintances. He taught us well about devotion and courage. As his life ebbed, Barry took extra precautions to lessen our sorrow and to encourage us to enter into fellowship with one another. He made certain that we paid close attention. "I'm going to teach you how to handle pain and despair."

The midnight blue and silver Freightliner is, no doubt, out on the highway somewhere, perhaps traversing Interstate 85 to Roanoke or Interstate 24 to St. Louis. Its memorial duties completed, it pulls trailers packed with television sets, lawn tractors, or supplies for fast food chains. Little boys and big boys will glance as it passes, hoping for a response as they signal its driver with a raised arm for a honk on its powerful air horn. For me this soulful sound will forever evoke a memory of Barry Walker, who rests in peace.

SOURCES AND ACKNOWLEDGMENTS

I am grateful to Barry's parents, Leon and Carolyn Walker, his brother, Parrish, and his sister, LeAnne, for generously sharing their memories and photographs with me.

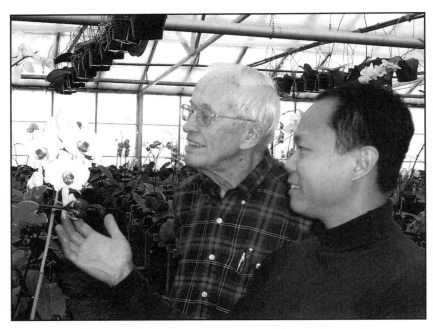

Hat Chau (right) and John Lines, owner of the greenhouse where
Hat works and propagator of a unique species of orchid named for Hat.

THE ORCHID GROWER:
HAT CHAU

—⟨∿⟩—

From the glass-enclosed office on the sixth floor, we were treated to a beautiful twilight. The November sun cast a warm yellow glow over Missionary Ridge to our east, and clouds at the horizon caught a rosy cast from the west before fading into violet. The hues reminded me of the orchids that my friend cultivated. Both of us were fatigued, Hat from his work at the greenhouse, me from a particularly busy Friday's clinic. During a twelve-year interval, I had gathered snatches of the lives of Hat and his father in Cambodia, and I knew that each fragment of history evoked painful memories for Hat. He promised someday to tell me his story sequentially. That day had arrived.

Hat Chau's world had disintegrated in 1975 when he was seven years old. He and his family — Father Heng, Mother Kon, three older sisters, an older brother, and two younger brothers — lived in the Cambodian village of Chomnon, close to the border with Thailand. Heng worked as an agricultural middleman, purchasing rice from farmers and finishing the grain before transporting it to the cities for sale. Heng tended toward Chinese religious traditions of reverence for ancestors; Kon worshipped at the village's Buddhist shrine. Hat had just one year of school behind him when the Communist Khmer Rouge forces began their relentless drive through the countryside. To escape them, Heng moved his family to

Battembang, a nearby city under firm government control, where he had relatives. For a few months the Chau family lived securely in an apartment, but the noose of the insurgents gradually tightened around the city until one day soldiers and police vanished. Military trucks carrying sullen-faced troops dressed in ragged uniforms rolled over city streets.

"I was scared. Something was not right. Something terrible was going to happen," Hat recalls.

The Khmer Rouge closed all markets, shops, and banks. The national currency collapsed. Residents tried to protect their possessions but quickly had to barter these for food. For a few days quiet prevailed; perhaps life would not be so bad after all, everyone hoped. Then with no warning, Khmer Rouge soldiers spread throughout all the neighborhoods, firing their weapons into the air, ordering everyone to leave the city. Parents tried desperately to locate children who had gone to playgrounds or to run errands. Children returned to empty houses whose adults had already been driven away. Screams and cries of separated families echoed through the streets as soldiers forced everyone into the countryside. Within three hours the city was empty. Most evacuees escaped with only a single pack containing a few items of clothing, some water, and a few handfuls of rice. Many families sought in vain to find missing children.

Heng Chau had been able to gather his entire family outside the city. Having nowhere else to go, he led his wife and children on a two-day walk to their village. They arrived at a scene of complete desolation. Guerillas had sacked and burned most houses, destroyed gardens and rice crops, and killed all livestock. Hat and his family scoured nearby fields for precious grains of rice. A few days lapsed before Khmer Rouge soldiers returned to the village, establishing strict curfews and arbitrary restrictions on movement and commerce. On the morning of the second day of occupation, soldiers ordered all children to muster in the center of the village. With no time for farewells, the soldiers marched the children away from the village, dividing them among forced labor camps two or more days march away. The soldiers made certain that no siblings would serve in the same camp.

Four years would pass before Hat Chau would again see a member of his family. His parents and his youngest brother, who was four years old, remained in the village. They received no information regarding the location or fate of their abducted family members.

* * *

Cambodia occupies the southwest corner of the Indochinese Peninsula. Viet Nam borders on the east, Laos on the north, and Thailand on the west and northwest. A coastline of two hundred miles opens onto the Gulf of Thailand. The nation is approximately the size of Missouri. Emerging from French oversight after France's defeat in the Indochina War of 1953, at first Cambodia enjoyed relative stability under the leadership of Prince Norodom Sihanouk, who was able to suppress the Communist guerrilla forces (the Khmer Rouge) led by Pol Pot, a vicious, radical leader. Prince Sihanouk maintained a delicate balancing act among various national and international forces. Though technically neutral, Cambodia appeared to the United States government to be overly sympathetic to China and North Viet Nam.

Cambodia could not escape involvement in the Viet Nam war. Geography made Cambodia an ideal supply route for troops and supplies from North Viet Nam to South Viet Nam. In an attempt to drive the North Vietnamese from Cambodia, American-led forces invaded Cambodia in 1970. That same year the forces of Pol Pot staged a sucessful military coup and overthrew Prince Sihanouk, relentlessly extending their control over rural areas in the western portion of the nation. Khmer Rouge efforts were abetted by the fierce bombardment from American aircraft in 1973; the Communist forces within Cambodia opposed a peace treaty that would end fighting on the Indochina Peninsula. Another massive air attack tipped support of the peasantry to Pol Pot. One by one besieged cities, such as Battembang, fell to the Khmer Rouge.

In American eyes Cambodia represented a footnote to larger events in neighboring Viet Nam. A coup or confrontation seemed always underway among democratic forces, the army, supporters of Prince Sihanouk (who was briefly returned to power under the Pol Pot regime), and various Communist factions. The United States suffered battle fatigue and urgently sought disengagement from the Viet Nam War. The invasion and aerial bombardment of Cambodia hastened that disengagement, and I do not recall great opposition to either in the American media or in public debate. The attitude seemed to be that if Cambodia had to be destroyed so that United States troops could be extricated from Viet Nam, then so be it.

Pol Pot believed that city life corrupted its citizens, who could only be purified by agricultural work in the countryside. He ordered the relocation of nearly all urban dwellers to forced labor camps. City life and business ceased. The right of private ownership of property was abolished. An estimated one million of Cambodia's seven million people perished in the abrupt, brutal dislocations, from starvation and disease, or at the hands of roving death squads of Khmer Rouge executioners.

When Vietnamese forces invaded Cambodia in 1979, they slowly wrested the tortured nation from the grips of the cruel and twisted Pol Pot. By 1990 Cambodia had regained a measure of self-rule.

★   ★   ★

Hat estimates the age range of the children enslaved with him at six to fourteen years. The children worked without a day of rest from sunrise to sunset, cultivating rice paddies, building dykes, and digging irrigation ditches. The soldiers forced the children to march everywhere they went. The rags that covered their bodies stayed constantly damp from sweat and the water of the rice patties. They never had adequate food or water. As far as Hat observed, neither a physician nor a nurse ever visited his camp. Sick children either died or somehow managed to drag their bodies to the day's work detail. Hat witnessed burial details as they dug shallow graves in the forests into which they tossed emaciated bodies, which they hurriedly covered with dirt. If a child-worker was observed to slacken his efforts, he or she would be whipped and humiliated in the evenings in the presence of coworkers.

"They had no parents, no one to comfort them. Many children died. They cried out for parents who were not there. They died of heartache."

I asked how he had managed to survive.

"I tried not to think about what I was doing. I tried to look at the fields or the sky and find something beautiful to think about. This was hell on earth. I had a strong will to live. I had to see this to the end. God is a God of justice. Sometimes we have to wait."

Nighttime provided little rest for the children. They slept on cots made of roughly split bamboo strips that had been lashed together with cord. No straw mats or bedclothes softened their beds. The thatched or tin roofs they lay beneath leaked copiously during monsoon rains. They received no schooling, only occasional lectures in political doctrine. All religious practices were banned.

Hat lost track of time as one relentless day followed another for four years, until 1979. As the guards seemed to grow increasingly uneasy, Hat overheard rumors that the Vietnamese army had invaded Cambodia. Then one day the Khmer Rouge troops abruptly disappeared, seeking to escape into the forests. Those children who were strong enough to walk immediately left the camp in search of their homes and their families.

Hat had always possessed a remarkable sense of direction. Hungry and thirsty, he nevertheless managed to reach his village after a walk of several days. Afraid of being captured, he walked at night and rested during the hours of daylight. Remarkably, all of his dispersed siblings found their way home during the next several weeks.

Hat learned that his mother had died. Adults of the village had been forced into brutal routines of labor, and Kon had became progressively weak. She was told to work or else, but she continued to weaken and eventually could not longer rise from her bed. Denied any treatment, she died several days later.

Heng and his children were uncertain as to what they should do or where they should go. They feared the resurgence of Khmer Rouge forces, and the village did not have sufficient food for its remaining occupants. All but two older daughters decided to leave, stealthily moving through dense forests to reach the border with Thailand after a hike of several days. Heng bribed a guard with his remaining resources to guide the family across an unmanned section of the border. A walk of an additional day brought the Chau family to a sprawling refugee camp. This would be home for two years.

Although the camp had the support of the Red Cross and other international relief agencies, there was never enough food or water. Tens of thousands of Cambodians occupied the tent city. Occasionally a class in reading was offered to the children. Hat remembers walking constantly along the twisting, narrow streets of the camp. The refugees shared a fear of being returned to Cambodia and the bestial Khmer Rouge. Uncertainty, crowding, and insufficient provisions spawned an atmosphere of intense anxiety and short tempers. The occupants of the camp assumed that a disaster lay just ahead. During his confinement within the camp, after seeing a film on the life of Christ, Hat converted to Christianity. "It made sense to me," he said. "The missionairies spoke of things that I felt."

Before long, Heng had formulated a bold plan for his family. They would emigrate to the United States. A paternal uncle had settled in California years earlier, and a brother-in-law resided in Chattanooga, Tennessee where he enjoyed the friendship of a very determined lady named Charlotte Harris. The application process to emigrate dragged on for months. Heng often waited for hours for an interview with an official before being told that he would have to return the next day. Officials lost or mislaid documents that had required hours to complete. No one in the camp's administrative hierarchy provided an encouraging word. Until Charlotte Harris.

Learning of the Chau family's plight from Heng's brother-in-law, Mrs. Harris, a widow, tackled the bureaucracy from the American side of the Pacific Ocean. She volunteered to serve as the family's sponsor. Months later the sluggish immigration system responded and issued visas for Heng, Hat, his two younger brothers, his oldest brother and his wife and two young children, and his oldest sister, enabling them all to leave Thailand for Signal Mountain, Tennessee, and the home of Charlotte Harris.

"She was like a second mother to me," Hat remembers. "I asked her once why she took us in. She told me she did it for the Lord and not for herself."

Charlotte Harris lived in a small house on the east brow of Signal Mountain. Her friends from church wondered how she could possibly accommodate within her modest home a family of nine who spoke no English and had no possessions beyond the clothing that they wore. She assured her friends that she and her Cambodian charges might be cramped for a while but would cope quite nicely. Her friends did not further question a lady whom they agreed was "formidable" whenever she directed her attention to any project, whether founding and lead-ing Girl Scout troops or directing children's choirs. They recall that Charlotte Harris had no interest in calling attention to her volunteer works for her community.

The Chau family lived with Charlotte Harris until an apartment could be located for them. Heng obtained work as an assistant in a garage. Hat began ninth grade at Signal Mountain Middle School in September 1984, his first formal education since being marched from his village nine years earlier. He spoke no English and had no idea what was being discussed in each class, so Charlotte Harris worked with him most evenings. She urged Hat to underline in his textbooks those words or sentences that he did not understand. Hat recalls underlining everything. Patiently, using gestures and pictures, Charlotte Harris opened Hat's mind to his new culture and language.

The next year, the family moved to nearby Rossville, Georgia. Now a confident student, Hat improved quickly in his studies, graduating from high school on schedule in 1988. He earned money to attend Hiawassee Junior College, gaining a diploma in business administration, before entering the University of Tennessee at Chattanooga. Hat worked a variety of gardening and landscaping jobs to pay for his tuition and books. In 1993 he earned his bachelor's degree in human resources management. By this time all of Hat's family save his father had moved to California. Charlotte Harris remained his friend and advisor until her death in 1996. He reveres her memory.

Hat began his first job with a landscaping company. Noticing how much the hardworking young Asian man enjoyed working with decorative plants, the company's foreman advised Hat to seek work at a nearby greenhouse that specialized in orchids. At Lines Orchids on Signal Mountain, Hat found the beauty that he had first sought in the fields and in the sky overlying the forced labor camp. When his father retired and moved to California to live with his eldest son, as Cambodian custom dictates, Hat chose to remain with the orchids. He wanted to learn how to grow and hybridize a variety of species. The orchids in their rich colors became the pigments on his palette. Outside of work, he landscaped the space in front of his dwelling, then contracted with other homeowners to transform their lawns and gardens into special places of beauty.

"Sometimes when I have no orchids or other plants to work with, I paint them on a piece of paper."

"How did you do it, Hat?" I asked. "How did you stay sane? How did you maintain your humanity during the dark years?"

"In the labor camp I thought over and over, 'This is not what life is all about. There has to be something beautiful beyond this.'"

"What do you worry about these days, Hat?"

"I worry about my youngest brother. He joined the Navy in 1985. I worry about him being in Iraq."

Night had fallen when we ended our conversation. Hat had brought an orchid, a white, purple-tinged Cattleya, for my wife. "Give this to Mrs. Cleaveland," he said as he presented it to me.

"It's beautiful," I replied.

"I know," responded Hat.

★　★　★

Children, then grandchildren, have brought happiness to me that I could not imagine before their arrival. I rejoice in their presence whether we are sharing a book, taking a hike, or visiting a playground. I delight in photographs of them, and in the photographs that patients show to me of their children and grandchildren. When five-year-old Lydia telephones an update of the activities of her new puppy, I listen attentively, my day immediately brightened. Seven-year-old Matthew proudly reports his designation as the "best sportsman" on his soccer team at a pizza party marking the end of a season in which they lost most of their games. Four-year-old Rachel, emulating a dog, chooses to answer my enquiries with yaps and barks. We are kept kinder, more honest, and more appreciative of the gifts of life when we are with children, either of our own family or the families of others. When I read of an instance of abuse of a child, I am stunned and saddened. Even if the adult abuser of a child is mentally ill or made wild by alcohol or drugs, I still have trouble understanding how he or she could hurt a child. Organized, widespread brutality to children, whether at the hands of an Adolf Hitler or a Pol Pot, staggers my senses and makes me question whether such monsters belong to some species other than *Homo sapiens*.

I can cope with my despair when I contemplate the gentle wisdom, the courage, and the indestructible belief of a Hat Chau that this earth is ultimately suffused with beauty. We may have to wait for it, but it will come.

SOURCES AND ACKNOWLEDGMENTS

The maps of Southeast Asia in the *National Geographic Atlas of the World* allowed me to trace events of the Indochina wars and the journeys of Hat Chau and his family. *When the War Was Over: Cambodia and the Khmer Rouge Revolution* (1986) by Elizabeth Becker refreshed my memories of that time and added new perspectives.

John Lines and Hat Chau gave me a tour of the greenhouses of Lines Orchids, surely one of the loveliest interiors on Earth.

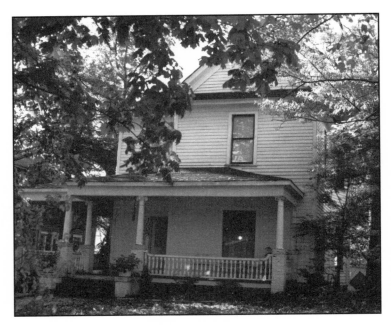

Marjorie Hardee's renovated house.

RENOVATIONS:
MARJORIE HARDEE

—⟿—

I checked the number on the house — 1005; it matched my directions, but something was amiss. The once elegant, two-storied house was in shambles and seemed deserted, an appropriate locale for a Halloween haunted house. Perhaps I had recorded the wrong number. Ten in the morning, coffee with the mother of our son's fiancée, a first meeting, but surely not in a wrecked house. Just then the screened front door opened and a voice hailed me. "You must be Clif. Excuse the mess. Just be careful."

Marjorie Hardee directed me along the temporary walkway that crossed the front porch and led into the entryway. She explained that termites had been hard at work at this site for years, and that all of the flooring and some of the supporting two by fours had to be ripped from the porch. Hardly had we shaken hands and completed our introductions than Marjorie had me in tow, touring the house that she had recently purchased. She assumed the role of project foreman. We peered around plastic sheeting that covered doorways. Already the floor finishers had begun the removal of layers of dark varnish to uncover the natural grain of oak planks. The dry wallers, meanwhile, were at work, steaming and peeling generations of paint and paper from the walls of each room. In some places duct tape covered ragged holes in the walls.

Marjorie explained that college students who had previously occupied the house had all but destroyed its interior. Some elegant features survived, hinting at the house's former life. She pointed out the crown molding in each room, the solid oak doors and window frames. Where she saw possibilities, I saw wreckage, imagining a succession of parties and impromptu indoor football games staged by the previous occupants.

Our tour completed, Marjorie brewed coffee for us in the shell that had been a kitchen. At this and every subsequent visit, she was the quintessential hostess, animated, welcoming, never letting conversation flag. She showed me detailed plans for the house's complete renovation. The work should be finished before the wedding of our children, she said. I silently doubted her optimism and wondered why Marjorie had not opted to demolish the house and build a new home on the attractive, tree-studded lot. Surely it would cost less money and aggravation than the complex task that lay before her. I understood neither Marjorie's ability to sense hidden beauty nor her determination to rescue this house from a wrecking ball. Masculine practicality conflicted with feminine aesthetics.

When the wedding of Karen Hardee and Rance Cleaveland rolled around, the house at 1005 Lamond Street became the epicenter for the festivities. Marjorie and her work crews had met their timelines and produced a gem. Most of the interior woodwork had been preserved and shone beneath clear varnish. The walls were flawless and smooth beneath mellow tones of blue, tan, and ivory. I marveled at the artistry of the original builders and the restorers of this seventy-five-year-old home. The house had been extensively restored yet seemed as if it had been lived in by its current owner for decades. Marjorie's love of her home could not have been greater had it been the ancestral wellspring of her family. She hosted lunches, dinners, drop-ins, and weekend stays of visiting friends, always quietly proud of her residence in Durham, North Carolina. Her neighbors and many friends dubbed her "The Queen of Lamond Street."

Fourteen years later, in the spring of 2002, Marjorie died in that house. Eight weeks earlier she had telephoned her children to tell them that she had widespread carcinoma. She wished to remain at home under the care of her physician and visiting nurses. Marjorie paused when her children asked how long she had been sick.

"I found out about four years ago," she responded.

A worsening cough, much deeper than the morning cough produced by her longtime consumption of cigarettes, had compelled Marjorie to consult her internist. An X-ray and a scan uncovered a malignant tumor in the center of her chest. Involvement of surrounding lymph nodes precluded surgery. Marjorie carefully considered options of radiation and chemotherapy before rejecting both. Her background in clinical nursing informed her decision. She feared that side-effects from such therapy would rob her of her independence and force her to leave her home. She did not want to become a burden for her children. Her physician honored Marjorie's choice and pledged to keep her comfortable. Marjorie elicited a further promise: she did not want anyone else, neither friend nor relative, to know that she had cancer.

"I don't want everyone pestering me, asking how I am feeling. I don't want to trouble the children."

Her physician agreed to this request.

Marjorie resumed her work at a nearby Ronald McDonald House. Her social schedule did not miss a beat. Medication suppressed her cough, and no one could recall evidence of sadness during her subsequent years. The "Queen" shared photographs and news of her grandchildren with the parade of visitors to her home. In 2000 she reduced her work hours, and in 2001 she helped care for Karen as she recovered from serious surgery. In the spring of 2002, a tumor that had lain remarkably dormant in Marjorie's chest exploded into widespread, painful metastases. It was then she called her children and notified her friends, who would share a bed-side vigil during the remaining weeks of her life. She quietly eased away one Saturday afternoon. A grandson closed her memorial service with the benediction, "Dear God, thank you for Grandma Marjorie."

Another story of pain and triumph remained to be told.

Marjorie was born in 1930 in Melbourne, Australia, the third of four daughters. From early childhood she entertained no other goal than becoming a nurse. She completed her training as a clinical "sister" at Prince Henry's College. Always ready for adventure and new sights, Marjorie accepted a job in London. No sooner had she boarded ship for England than she met Gilbert Hardee, a young American graduate student en route to Egypt. Their days afloat led to a romance. Within a year Marjorie traveled to the United States to marry Gilbert, who was completing his dissertation in rural sociology. A year later the couple departed for Iran where Gilbert would conduct research in family planning. His career would be devoted to the design and implementation of programs for birth control in impoverished Asian communities.

Donna Hardee was born in Iran. At the conclusion of Gilbert's two-year assignment, the family faced a dilemma. Should they remain in Iran where Gilbert had offers of work from international agencies or should they return to America where he had offers to join university faculties? They chose the latter option. Gilbert joined the faculty at North Carolina State University in Raleigh where the family would spend the next seven years, during which Jeff and Karen were born.

Gilbert and Marjorie could not shake their love of travel and life in foreign cultures. When the United States Agency for International Development proffered a job in Asia, Gilbert accepted at once with Marjorie's enthusiastic endorsement. In a succession of assignments in the Philippines, Pakistan, Nepal, and Malaysia, Gilbert worked exhaustively to promote humane family planning in cultures stressed by soaring populations, rising poverty, and diminishing natural resources.

After a tour in Manila, the Hardees moved to Katmandu, Nepal, which was Marjorie's favorite of all of her family's assignments. She served as a volunteer nurse in a large orphanage. Karen, then six years old, often accompanied her mother to work. Karen recalls the absolute stillness of the children while the Anglo woman in a white dress moved among them. Marjorie spoke of a special mission in caring for children who had so little hope. The orphans were the point toward which she felt her life had been aimed.

An assignment to Pakistan followed. The pattern of relocation did not vary. Upon receiving new orders, Marjorie directed the packing of personal possessions, which typically would not reach their next destination until weeks, even months, after the family's arrival. Even in the temporary absence of her furniture, Marjorie energetically set out to convert every one of the family's habitats into a home.

In each setting the Hardees considered themselves "cultural Christians," observing within their circle of Western expatriates the major religious holidays but seldom attending church services otherwise. The later lives of the children suggest that they paid close attention to the lessons presented during the major celebrations of the church.

The family lived in Karachi while Gilbert traveled widely in the country, split at that time into a western section that constitutes present-day Pakistan and an eastern section that would become Bangladesh. Local regulations prevented Marjorie from obtaining a work-permit and, restless, she began a pattern of excessive alcohol consumption at the frequent social events hosted by members of the western enclave.

A subsequent posting to Kuala Lumpur, the capital of Malaysia, would nearly prove fatal for Marjorie. Books and other cherished belongings were extensively damaged in shipment. Gilbert's work kept him away from home for weeks at a time. Marjorie found few friends in an expatriate community dominated by commercial delegations. She retreated to her bed for days at a time, remaining in an alcohol and tranquillizer-induced fog. She lost weight and seemed increasingly agitated when awake. Her children feared that she would soon die. They finally convinced her to see a physician who diagnosed hyper-thyroidism. Although medication reversed her weight loss and stemmed her agitation, Marjorie remained addicted to alcohol and be-came dependent as well upon Valium, which had been prescribed as part of the therapy for her overactive thyroid. Gilbert implored Mar-jorie to seek medical treatment in Australia where she could convalesce in the company of her family, but she declined.

"It broke Dad's heart. She wouldn't let us help her," remembers Karen.

★　　★　　★

Half a world away, I worked my half-day assignments in the depen-dents' clinic at Ireland Army Hospital at Fort Knox. The base provided advanced armor training for young soldiers who were destined for duty in Viet Nam. Returning troops carried stories of the vulnerability of our tanks and armored personnel carriers in the war zone. In a context of dread and inevitability, a surprising number of spouses of trainees devel-oped sudden severe hyperthyroidism. Weight loss, heat intolerance, nervousness — the triad of symptoms became quite familiar to those of us assigned to care for the soldiers' families. We could treat the disease but not the cause. In subsequent years of clinical practice, I continue to see occasional instances in women where sustained and seemingly insolvable stress stimulates severe over-activity of the thyroid gland. Marjorie Hardee had become entrapped in her own personal theater of combat.

★   ★   ★

Marjorie rallied during a furlough with her family in the United States before embarking upon a fresh assignment in Islamabad. Donna and then Jeff departed for college in America. For a time Marjorie seemed at peace among her friends in the foreign-aid community. While Gilbert worked an especially demanding schedule, Marjorie accepted a series of volunteer nursing responsibilities, which she found challenging and enjoyable. Unfortunately, while in Islamabad Gilbert suffered a mild heart attack. His convalescence would bring a welcome return to America, just in time to celebrate Thanksgiving of 1976.

Gilbert, Marjorie, and Karen arrived at an apartment in Michigan where Donna and Jeff attended college. This would serve as their temporary home. Soon after they had unpacked, however, Gilbert was felled by a severe heart attack. He died hours later.

"Mom collapsed within herself," Donna recalls.

Marjorie fell into a depression of such severity that no one could penetrate it. Her children became of necessity her guardians and care-givers. Five times Marjorie would attempt suicide.

Karen remembers that interval. "The four years between Dad's death and Mom's emergence from her severe depression and suicide attempts were absolute hell for all of us."

With their sole possessions contained in their suitcases (the family's belongings would not arrive from Islamabad for months), the children decided they and their mother would live in Raleigh, North Carolina, the last place they had lived before beginning their overseas odyssey. The move meant that Donna and Jeff would have to interrupt their college educations and that Karen would not be able to rejoin her senior high school class at the international school in Islamabad. The Hardees had maintained close ties with friends from Gilbert's tenure at North Carolina

State University. These friends would repeatedly demonstrate their love for the Hardee family in the painful months that followed.

Once, in an attempt at abstinence, Marjorie ceased drinking abruptly and suffered delirium tremens, for which she was hospitalized. The Carolina friends worked tirelessly alongside her children to keep Marjorie sober and alive. Cycles of heavy drinking, prescribed tranquillizers, inpatient and outpatient psychiatric treatment and electroconvulsive shock therapy ensued. Brief improvements in Marjorie's health were followed by severe reversals. A sister came from Australia to assist in Marjorie's care, and close friends provided homes for Donna, Jeff, and Karen, who sensed that soon they would be orphaned.

Marjorie took an overdose of medication, then another and another. Ironically, each time Marjorie exited a psychiatric hospital, she had fresh prescriptions for a variety of tranquillizers and antidepressants, the materials for the next attempt on her life. A succession of physicians relinquished efforts to assuage her despair, but her children refused to give up, even though Marjorie in her present state bore little resemblance to the mother of their earlier years.

As the first anniversary of Gilbert's death neared, Marjorie appeared to achieve sobriety. Jeff returned to college, and Karen matriculated at nearby Duke University. Donna remained with Marjorie. But a final calamity lurked just ahead.

Somehow Marjorie had obtained a shotgun. Perhaps this was her final safeguard against a relapse into alcoholism. Possibly alcohol represented a delaying action until she could achieve a final solution for her overwhelming grief. On a morning that had seemed calm and routine, she removed her weapon from its hiding place and in the woods behind her house delivered a single blast to her abdomen. Hearing the report and surmising its cause, Donna ran to the aid of her mother. Miraculously, Marjorie survived, but many weeks would pass before she emerged from danger. While taking turns at her bedside, Donna, Jeff, and Karen assumed management of the family's shrinking resources. In the months that followed, Marjorie continued to gain strength.

After she had recovered from the gunshot wound, Marjorie purchased a house in Raleigh. She considered options for resuming her work in nursing, yet she could not free herself from a lingering despair. She decided to sell her home and travel to Australia, thinking that time with her family in her native land might dissipate her sadness. She gauged correctly.

Marjorie's family urged her to remain longer in Australia. Though still emotionally shaky from her recent wound, Marjorie elected to return to America; her children defined home for her. During her return journey, Jeff suffered extensive injuries in an accident at college. Upon reaching America, Marjorie directed her energies to his recovery. The person whose life had been consumed by alcohol and tranquillizers had been buried, and a resolute woman now occupied her place.

"Our mother had returned," Donna reflects.

Jeff finished college, married, and began a business career that would eventually take him to Singapore. Donna completed ministerial studies in preparation for a career in foreign missions. Karen completed her doctoral studies in family planning. Marjorie seemed happy in administrative work at a hotel outside Durham, and she began a search for a place that she could transform into a home. She became captivated with the possibilities presented by an abandoned house on Lamond Street in Durham. The rehabilitation of the structure dominated her thoughts and activities, and after six months the beautifully renovated home welcomed family and guests in the days preceding Karen's marriage to Rance Cleaveland in the Duke Chapel. The Hardee family was again secure.

When a Ronald McDonald House opened in Durham, Marjorie accepted a position that she cherished, seeing to the needs of pediatric patients and their families who had come to Duke Medical Center for treatment of malignant disorders. In many respects this job recalled the special experience of working with orphans in Nepal. A lifelong calling had been redefined and followed.

★   ★   ★

My father-in-law, Bill Pfeffer, raised Angus cattle, corn, and soy beans in southern Illinois. Father of three young children, he lost his right arm in a shooting accident in 1940. Within three weeks he returned to his work on the farm. Throughout his farming career, he had an eye for wood. When old farm houses in his community were being razed, he visited the sites in search of wood panels and boards that otherwise would be burned or hauled to dumps. Many of the houses had featured interiors of walnut, cherry, oak, and ash. Somehow, through the overlying grime and splintered surfaces, Bill discerned swirls of natural grain, features that he could visualize in furniture that he planned one day to make. When age dictated Bill's retirement from farming, he applied his energies to woodworking, setting up an elaborate array of braces, clamps, and pulleys that would allow a one-armed man to saw, plane, rout, and finish. He produced for his children and grandchildren end tables, coffee tables, buffets, china cabinets, and full-sized dinner tables. He was so prolific that I jokingly accused him once of harboring unpaid assistants within his shop.

Once, during a visit to his basement shop, my wife Ruzha and I rummaged through a stack of dusty, splintered boards. Bill joined us. Ruzha picked up and examined an irregular piece of wood, four feet long, eight inches at its widest, whose shape suggested a fish. Bark adhered to one edge; a deep, black gouge marked one end; the other end seemed to have been charred. Bill recalled pulling the plank from a smoldering pyre.

"Look at that grain." He used a rag to brush dirt from the surface.

Ruzha nodded; she saw what her dad had perceived. I still saw a grimy, rough-surfaced board. "If you like it," he said, "I'll finish it for you." Trusting that Bill saw something in the wood that I could not, I replied that I liked it.

Months later, during another visit to the Pfeffer farm, Bill gave me my "fish," a splendidly finished piece of cherry. Bark delineated its upper edge. The darkened gouge suggested an eye; the charred end had become a tail. The piece hangs above a sideboard, also made by Bill, in our dining room. I am amazed each time I contemplate Bill's gift. It triggers immediate memories of a courageous man who refused a label of "handicapped" and who could look deeply into damaged wood to perceive beauty overlooked or not understood by the rest of us.

★   ★   ★

Marjorie Hardee's children and closest friends remembered the beauty that infused her spirit. They refused to surrender her to a grief of such intensity that it defied all available therapies. Stubborness, prayer, and love brought Marjorie to safety, and she lived twenty full years after her final, nearly fatal, suicide attempt, years that her children never thought they would see. Marjorie cherished these years, finally at home with herself and her life, restored as lovingly as she had restored the house at 1005 Lamond Street. For Marjorie, these years would witness the launching of her children's internationally oriented careers, the birth of five grandchildren, and the establishment of a place that she would call "home."

When confronted with someone, a loved one perhaps or a stranger, who is in the prolonged throes of despondency, alcoholism, and drug addiction, the question arises as to how long we should persist in trying to rescue them. Donna, Jeff, and Karen Hardee answered "forever, if necessary." They succeeded after a grueling fight on their mother's behalf. I have known other families who simply became so exhausted in trying to bring a loved one to safety in similar circumstances that they could go no further. Their loved one ended up dead, in long-term institutional care, or sustained in a drug-induced daze by caregivers who have found no other option for therapy. On other occasions, I have seen families who mounted efforts similar to the Hardee children, yet still lost their loved one to suicide or cirrhosis. I believe that the majority of people in circumstances similar to those of Marjorie Hardee do not survive their illnesses.

So what determines survivorship? Donna Hardee attributes her mother's survival to prayer, a belief that I share. But what are the implications of a death that occurs despite devoutly rendered prayers for recovery? Does that mean that the prayers were somehow faulty or that God was not listening at the moment the prayers were rendered? I believe that all prayers are answered, but not necessarily in ways that we may recognize. Prayer may steel family and friends of a deeply troubled person to stay the course even when they are exhausted. Prayer may make a grief bearable if the stricken person dies. Prayer may clarify seemingly chaotic or contradictory conditions and open up fresh possibilities for thought and action. Prayer certainly links those who cherish a severely troubled person into a team capable of providing far more support than the strongest individual can muster.

Finally, prayer brings courageous behavior into the reach of all of us.

I can close my eyes and visualize a miracle of healing that was built one tough day at a time. Bill Pfeffer could see beauty where others saw damaged wood. Even more wonderfully, three brave children saw possibilities in their beloved mother that eluded others.

SOURCES AND ACKNOWLEDGMENTS

I am grateful to Donna and Karen Hardee for their candor and patience in sharing with me the story of their mother.

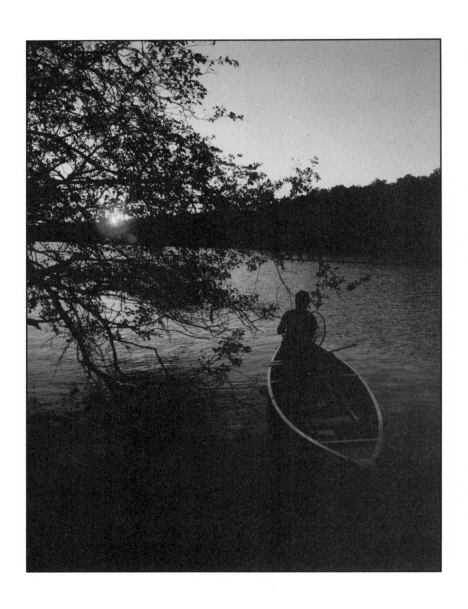

FIFTY YEARS ON

—◦◦◦—

We met fifty years ago at summer camp. My job as handyman at the Girl Scout camp fit nicely into the few months that preceded my entry into college. The pay was reasonable, certainly better than the fifty cents an hour I had earned during the previous summer as a cashier at a service station. I knew the director and many of the counselors from my years in LaGrange, so the job represented a reunion of sorts. Three males — two college students from Mississippi and I — were hired for such varied jobs as tending the stable of four horses, repairing anything that broke, running errands in the camp station wagon, and investigating any after-hours noises.

Six weeklong camp sessions took place on the shores of a lake in the Roosevelt State Park in West Georgia, near the Warm Springs retreat of the late President. Campers arrived and departed on Sunday afternoons. Scouts were assigned twelve to a cabin under the supervision of counselors who were high school and college students. Older campers had the option of staying in four-person tents. Cabins and tents were clustered a brisk walk away from a large hall that encompassed the kitchen, storage rooms, and dining and assembly areas. A cabin fifty yards away and on the other side of the hall provided a room at one end for the camp's two cooks — two women of indeterminate age — and at the other end, space for the three handymen. The cooks listened to gospel music on their radio, while we listened to baseball games. Our agreeably hard work left us tired but never so fatigued that we could not stay awake until the final out.

With piles of fried chicken and an array of desserts, Sunday lunch represented the culinary high point of each week. Preparation for the feast usually kept the cooks busy until quite late on Saturday night. On the second Saturday evening of camp, long after the campers had retired and before the conclusion of the nightly baseball broadcast, roaring voices and clatter were heard from the kitchen. Upon entering, we found the two cooks, both inebriated, singing as they rolled out biscuit dough. One of the ladies had stripped to her waist; flour covered her arms and torso. Her companion offered us a drink from a pint Mason jar. Our arrival preceded that of the camp director by only a couple of minutes. After a verbal roasting, she banished the cooks to their quarters. The director and her staff finished the preparations for the next day's lunch. The cooks returned to work a day later upon giving pledges of sobriety, at least for the remainder of the camp session.

A camp identical to ours faced us across the half-mile-wide lake. Boy Scouts occupied the camp for the first two weeks of our tenure. Their routines of swimming, canoeing, and staging lakefront campfires mirrored that of our camp. A quite different group of teenaged boy and girl campers followed the Boy Scouts. From our swimming dock, we could see that the sexes carried out their waterfront activities at separate times. Boys wore T-shirts with their swimming trunks. Girls appeared at the lake in long robes that they removed to reveal black swimsuits extending to their knees and elbows. Curious counselors at our waterfront passed around a pair of binoculars to inspect these swimmers, who seemed displaced from an earlier century. At night a jumble of loud noise, a mixture of music and shouting, echoed across the lake from their camp.

One evening at midweek, four of us, two handymen and two counselors, decided to investigate a particularly noisy night at the other camp. We finished our cleanup work after a campfire session before setting out in two canoes. A quarter moon provided our only light.

Paddling silently across the lake, we beached our canoes in the shadows at one end of the swimming area. We stayed at the fringe of the woods as we stealthily made our way to the central hall where the increasing clamor originated. Everyone was inside. We crept closer until we could view the activities through the open double door and large screened windows at the rear of the lodge. An older man stood in front, swaying and loudly singing and chanting non-words. Boys and girls emulated their leader. Several people thumped tambourines. Suddenly a boy picked up a chair and hurled it against a wall. Others of the congregation upended the heavy benches that were scattered about the room. Here and there a young person sank to the floor.

Sylvia, one of the counselors, tugged at my sleeve.

"Let's get out of here," she whispered. She voiced what all of us no doubt felt. We quickly retreated to our canoes and paddled back across the lake. Sylvia left immediately for her cabin, while the remaining threesome tried to make some sense of what we had witnessed. We concluded that we had spied upon some sort of religious observance that to us had seemed to be spinning out of control. We had heard the term "holy-rollers" with no insight into its possible meaning. Perhaps we had just witnessed such worshippers in action. The noise continued well after we left our lakefront.

Sylvia was two years my senior, soon to be a junior at her university. We met on the first day that counselors arrived to prepare the camp for its opening. Thereafter we exchanged greetings and brief comments in the course of most days. Our only conversation before our paddle across the lake had occurred when I repaired a torn screen on her cabin door. We chatted amiably while I measured and cut screening and then tacked it into place. I do not think we ventured beyond basic biographical information and observations of camp routines. She had the sophistication and nonchalance that I associated with college coeds generally.

At breakfast on the morning after our cross-lake adventure, Sylvia appeared exhausted and distracted. Her brown hair had not been combed, and she seemed thrown together in contrast to her usual neatness. After breakfast she approached me to ask if there was a time when we might talk. It was my turn to drive into nearby Chipley to pick up mail and supplies and browse the farmers' market for peaches and watermelons, so Sylvia obtained permission to join me, stating that she needed to place a phone call and to buy some personal items.

As I steered the station wagon along the twin-rutted road to the paved state highway, Sylvia began. "It was horrible; it was just horrible. How could they do that?"

I glanced at her. Tears streaked her cheeks. I asked if I there was anything I could do to help. She asked if I believed in hell, and in my fallen-Baptist state I replied that I did not know but I suspected that an all-loving God would not create such a place. She told me she believed in hellfire and damnation and further stated that she was doomed to reside in hell for eternity.

A master of the Cheerful Cliché, I offered up the notion that this could not be: we were all God's children. She was obviously kind and infinitely patient in working with children. Sylvia sobbed. Not knowing what else to do, I kept quiet and paid closer attention to my driving. Sylvia seemed composed by the time we reached Chipley.

Chipley would soon change its name to Pine Mountain and serve as the gateway town for Callaway Gardens, a recreational complex of golf courses, lakes, and scenic drives. Then, the tiny town had no public telephones. Long distance calls required a visit to the telephone exchange, a switchboard in the front bedroom of a private home. I waited while the owner-operator made the connection for Sylvia. I did not know whom she called, but I guessed that the attentiveness of the operator ensured that few secrets of the town's residents would escape her.

We completed our chores in town before visiting a roadside market to purchase fruit and melons for the camp. I thumped the large striped watermelons, testing them for ripeness, imitating a ritual that I had seen performed by all of the older males in my family. Unlike them, I thumped on faith, having no idea what sound signified ripeness. I purchased a dozen of the dark green melons and a bushel of peaches.

We began our return drive. Sylvia looked straight ahead. "I am a terrible person. I've done horrible things," she said.

She spoke vaguely of a discovery that a young boy had made in a vacation trailer, something about a man and a girl. She seemed to feel responsible. When I asked if she had ever discussed her worries with her parents, she fired a glance of incredulity at me. I sensed that I should remain quiet.

"You don't understand," she said to me. "You can't understand." She said nothing further before our return to camp.

★　★　★

In the 1950s my peers and I had a very limited emotional vocabulary and few resources for sorting out our troubles. I do not recall ever hearing terms such as "depression" or "anxiety." A "nervous breakdown" was a calamitous event that could hit a person like a bolt of lightning. We had no idea how to articulate our feelings or where we might seek help for emotional stresses. Schools had nurses who could check a temperature and determine who might need to go home or to see a doctor, but we would never seek counsel from them. These were kindly older women who would be shocked if we spoke of doubts or fears. Nor would we seek counsel from our family physicians, who had far more important work to accomplish than to listen to our worries. If we hinted to our parents that we had uncertainties about anything, we received a standard response: "Take it to the Lord in prayer." I prayed a lot, as did most of my friends, but I never received the clear and unequivocal answers I sought.

The church of that day had not defined its mission of counseling. It especially had no response to the raging hormones of adolescence. A revivalist once prayed before my high school Sunday school class, "Tear lust from our hearts." I recall touching my chest, possibly to determine if my heart was still in place. We did not dare raise sexual issues with our pastors or our Sunday school teachers. They would think that we were beyond redemption.

Parents and children of that day existed on opposite sides of a psychological divide. We were clothed, fed, and seemingly cherished, but we were also regarded as "little people" who would have to solve most problems of a non-physical nature on their own.

Nor did we as children, adolescents, or college students know how to ask our friends for help. Image was everything. A personal problem reflected weakness. Thus we kept our own counsel. When that proved inadequate, we took the edge off our grief and apprehension with beer.

★   ★   ★

I sensed Sylvia's distress, and I shared her helplessness, but I did not know how to respond to her plaints.

Counselors and staff enjoyed one evening a week off. Usually, several of us drove to nearby Columbus for supper and a movie. Sylvia rearranged her schedule to join four other counselors and me on our excursion to the city later in the week. We swapped jokes and stories over hamburgers and french fries before attending a forgettable Western with its forced, sappy ending. Sylvia sat next to me. As soon as the lights dimmed, she grasped my hand tightly and held it for the duration of the movie, releasing it only when the movie's credits rolled. As we walked to our station wagon, I paused with Sylvia while she studied clothing displayed in the shop's window.

"Thank you for listening. But, please, never tell anyone what I told you."

I was puzzled. I was not aware that I had been told anything that I could interpret, but I gave her my promise.

The remaining weeks of camp passed uneventfully. Sylvia occasionally aimed smiles at me, and we exchanged comments on the weather — very hot and humid — and the day's activities. After the departure of the final group of Scouts, staff remained for a day to pack gear and restore the premises to their former condition. Sylvia assisted while I tidied up the waterfront.

"Nothing is really wrong. Nothing happened. Forget that we ever spoke." We exchanged addresses before vacating the camp.

Later that year, I received a Christmas card from Sylvia and sent one in return. She jotted a note that all was well. The following spring she wrote at length, a long and rambling letter that reminisced about our experiences at camp. She recalled a statement of mine regarding our good fortune to be alive and well in such wonderful times. She challenged my optimistic musing. She alluded to her younger brother who suffered because he had once come unexpectedly upon his father and a girl as they embraced. The discovery had been a source of unending pain for her brother, although the event had occurred years earlier. She did know how to comfort him. A vague question formed in my mind. Could Sylvia have been the girl? I dismissed the notion at once. Fathers simply did not — could not — have romantic involvements with their daughters. Fathers might beat their children but never seduce them.

We continued our yearly exchange of Christmas greetings. She signed all of her correspondence, "Your wacky friend, Sylvia." I mailed a book to Sylvia upon her graduation from her university. In her response she outlined her plans to work in Atlanta while taking graduate courses. At Christmas time during my senior year, I traveled to Atlanta for interviews associated with a scholarship competition. Sylvia had mentioned the name of her employer in her Christmas card, so I called the company upon reaching Atlanta; she answered. She served as the firm's receptionist. Yes, she could meet me for lunch. Because she had but an hour we should meet in the dinette on the first floor of her office building.

Except for glasses and longer hair, she had not changed. We summarized our experiences of the past year and then ate in a companionable silence. Sylvia then spoke of a boy friend. They had dated most of the past year. He was a law student. He had repeatedly discussed the possibility of marriage after his graduation.

"I could never marry," she said.

"Why not?" I asked her.

"Not after everything that has happened. I could never marry him or anyone else."

I did not understand. In December 1957, the goals of young women I knew routinely included marriage and motherhood. When I pressed my question, Sylvia became teary and said that she had to return to work. Once again she had left me puzzled.

On a Sunday afternoon in the winter of 1960 in my Oxford boarding house, I was cramming for an examination in neuroanatomy. I had perfected a series of mnemonics for the name, location, and function of the twelve cranial nerves, and just as I began my final review, my landlady knocked at my door. Two women from the United States waited for me in the hallway downstairs. To my amazement, Sylvia and a traveling companion had called. She had saved my address from my last Christmas card.

The twosome had embarked upon a lengthy Grand Tour of western Europe. I forgot about anatomy so that I might guide them on a walking tour of Oxford capped by Evensong in the chapel of my college. Over supper Sylvia spoke of her relief at giving up a job that had become tedious. Upon her return from her vacation she planned to move to Washington, D.C. for employment that she had not yet identified. Her companion assured her that numerous employment opportunities existed in the District.

"How about your boy friend?" I asked.

Sylvia smiled. They were still friends but that was as far as the relationship would ever go. I spoke of my plans for marriage later in the year and how my wife and I would spend our first year in Oxford. When we parted, I extended a hand to Sylvia; she surprised me with a hug.

Several days later, I received a pale blue air letter from Sylvia. She and her friend had reached Paris and had viewed the city from atop the Eiffel Tower. She wrote that pressures from her job and from her suitor who pressed his proposals for marriage had overwhelmed her. She could cope only by closing the Atlanta chapter of her life. She wondered if she had not had "a nervous breakdown." She closed with her familiar salutation. I had no address to which I could respond until I received my annual card from Sylvia later in the year. She lived in the District of Columbia and felt contented in her job with a governmental agency.

We sustained our annual exchange of Yuletide greetings with brief updates of our lives. A decade passed. Sylvia's Christmas card carried a New Jersey address. She had married a teacher whom she had dated intermittently for several years. A later card reported the birth of a daughter. I telephoned my congratulations to her. As our conversation wound down, she recalled the broadly optimistic statement that I had made years earlier. She indicated that I was wrong, that life was difficult, and that she had to struggle at times to maintain her sanity. By that time I had been in medical practice for enough years to have insights into sadness that I had earlier lacked. I urged Sylvia to seek help from a psychiatrist or from her minister. She declined both suggestions. I offered to listen as a friend.

She declined this offer as well. "You would think your wacky friend was awful."

Years passed until one day I received a thick envelope from Sylvia, a letter of eight pages, four sheets front and back. Her handwriting had changed, no longer neat and aligned but irregular with drifting lines. She had ovarian carcinoma. The tumor had spread. After surgery, she had received chemotherapy. She had a lot of pain in her hip. She commented that her she had lost her hair and upbraided me again for my earlier optimism. She longed for happiness. She knew that her husband and daughter loved her but felt unworthy of their affection. She felt that she perpetrated a fraud each day, pretending to be someone that she was not. She spoke of her brother and his discovery so many years earlier. Her family had owned a small trailer that rested on riverfront property belonging to her parents. Her brother and one of his friends had hiked to the property one afternoon, and seeing the family's car alongside the trailer, her brother anticipated seeing his parents inside. He burst inside but just as quickly withdrew. He never spoke of what he had seen. He and his friend quickly retraced their several-mile route to their homes. That afternoon forever changed her family's life. She closed her letter:

"You must really think I'm crazy. Your wacky friend, Sylvia."

I telephoned her home. My call was redirected to the hospital. Sylvia told me that she felt in a fog because of medication she received. A minor fall had precipitated a fracture of her pelvis at the site of a metastasis, and she realized that she would soon die. She felt confident that her family had strength to deal with her loss. The hardest aspect of dying would be the loss of their companionship, she said. We joked about our camp experiences, recalling a time so far in the past that it seemed part of some ancestor's life. We spoke of our children and the good lives that we hoped they might have. I struggled to keep my voice steady. We said goodbye.

"God bless you, Clif," she said.

"God bless you, Sylvia."

Her husband sent me a copy of her obituary, which directed memorial contributions to her church.

★   ★   ★

I suspect that I am the sole repository of Sylvia's story. I never met another member of her family. I do not know if she had any siblings other than her younger brother. I never inquired of his situation. I suspect that Sylvia was the girl whom her brother had discovered in the arms of his father. I further suspect that there had been other sexual encounters between Sylvia and her father prior to the episode in the trailer. Alternatively, her brother might have found his father engaged in sexual intercourse with a friend of Sylvia's or some other young woman from the community, or a male. Her brother might then have told Sylvia what he had seen, and she did not know how to deal with the story and her brother's anguish. In yet another scenario, Sylvia might have been the discoverer. Whatever the scenario, the exposé at the trailer robbed Sylvia of serenity. She harbored a secret that would cast a pall over the remainder of her life, a secret that she could never articulate.

The chaotic religious service that Sylvia and I witnessed at the camp across the lake unleashed within her powerful recriminations. She felt responsible for whatever had happened. Despite college, a variety of jobs, a boy friend, a marriage, and the birth of her daughter, Sylvia labored to suppress a trauma that she could not assimilate. I do not know why she picked me as a comforter and a confidant. Possibly, I seemed safe and neutral and capable of maintaining a confidence. My handyman colleagues were too much in the mode of carefree fraternity boys. Sylvia had no close female friends among the camp's staff.

I wonder whom she telephoned in Chipley. The call may simply have been an excuse to get away from camp for a couple of hours and regain emotional control. Then and subsequently, I perhaps represented a safety valve for Sylvia, permitting her to subdue tumultuous memories for a time. I would like to think that had Sylvia consulted a psychiatrist and engaged in lengthy therapy, she could have found peace in her later life.

Sexual abuse within a family remains a complex tragedy that confers such guilt and helplessness upon its victims that they are loathe to seek assistance.

Despite her burdens, Sylvia trudged ahead. Suicide, a collapse into utter lassitude, alcoholism, or addiction to medication were possible outcomes that she was strong enough to reject. Her notes and letters form scattered points that I can only guess at connecting properly. For whatever reasons, she gave me glimpses of a life of grace and courage. My regret is that I did not know how to reach out in a fashion that might have helped her ease the burdens that she carried. I still have a picture of her, a photograph that she sent to me with a book of prayers to mark my graduation from college.

A HERO FOR
THE AGES
JANUSZ KORCZAK

*For the whole earth is the sepulcher of
famous men; and their story is not graven
only on stone over their native earth, but
lives on far away, without visible symbol,
woven into the stuff of other men's lives.
For you now it remains to rival what they
have done and, knowing the secret of
happiness to be freedom and the secret of
freedom a brave heart, not idly to stand
aside from the enemy's onset.*

THUCYDIDES, FROM THE
FUNERAL ORATION OF PERICLES

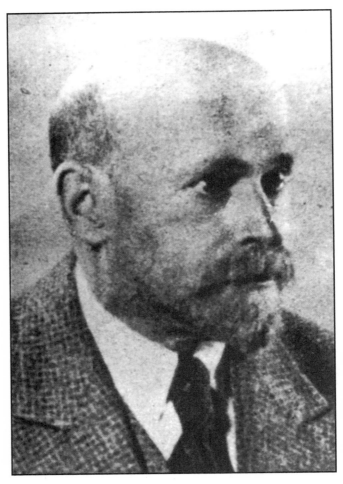

Janusz Korczak
(Photograph courtesy of the United States Holocaust
Memorial Museum.)

August 6, 1942, a hot and terrible day in the Warsaw Ghetto. Janusz Korczak, appearing frail and aged, walks in the front rank of a column of children. Colleagues of the Doctor bring up the rear. Worn and starving residents of the Ghetto watch from the sidewalks in silence as Nazi guards direct the procession toward the rail depot. For two years the Doctor and his staff have fought to keep these children alive in a Nazi-dominated hell. Now, all is lost. There can be no question that the distinguished physician and his companions on the forced march are destined for the death camp at Treblinka. No one panics. No one cries. Calmly the children follow their beloved guardian to the train station. He has prepared them for just such a moment.

★ ★ ★

Quite simply, Janusz Korczak is the most heroic figure that I know of. I first encountered Dr. Korczak in an article in the Sunday Magazine of *The New York Times* in 1980. Despite extensive readings in Holocaust literature, I had not previously noticed his name. The author of the article, Betty Jean Lifton, subsequently wrote a wonderful biography, *The King of Children: A Biography of Janusz Korczak,* in which the career of the pediatrician, philosopher, children's advocate, and hero of the Warsaw Ghetto is elegantly presented. I cannot overstate the inspirational value to me of her initial *Times* article and biography. Together they launched an on-going personal enquiry into the life and times of Janusz Korczak. My search has taken me repeatedly to the library of the United States Holocaust Memorial Museum with its poignant photographic archives, to bookstores and Web sites from which I have made too many purchases, and finally to Warsaw itself.

Janusz Korczak was not his birth name. Born in Warsaw in 1878 or 1879 he was named Henryk Goldszmit. Poland at the time was partitioned between Russia, Austria, and Prussia. Warsaw lay under control of the Czar. Henryk's paternal grandfather had been a surgeon. His father, Josef, had a distinguished career in law before mental illness forced his hospitalization for the final six years of his life. With this change in the family's fortunes, Henryk contributed to the support of his mother and younger sister by tutoring the children of affluent families. His authorial career began during these years with short pieces of fiction and nonfiction. He gained entry to medical school at Warsaw University. As a young medical student, he needed a penname for a literary competition. "Janusz Korczak" would gradually take the place of his real name.

Korczak's years of medical study were not confined to lecture halls, laboratories, and wards. He attended frequent meetings of the Peripatetic University, a free underground institute dedicated to socialist ideals and the preservation of Polish history and culture. He volunteered as a counselor for summer camps held in the countryside for impoverished Jewish children. He spent many evenings walking through the slums of Warsaw, learning firsthand of the plight of poor, malnourished children. He elicited their stories and became their confidant.

Upon completing his medical studies at Warsaw's Jewish Children's Hospital in 1905, Korczak began mandatory service in the Czarist army as a surgeon, assigned duty on a hospital train during Russia's war with Japan. At war's end, he returned to Warsaw to establish a private practice of pediatrics. While he had been away, his novel *Child of the Salon* had been serialized to wide acclaim. Twice he studied pediatrics abroad, spending a year in Berlin and several months in London and Paris. His parallel careers as writer and pediatrician flourished. In 1910 he astonished his patients and admirers by closing his practice to assume the directorship of a new orphanage for Jewish children.

Korczak's commitment to improving the welfare of children finds its most powerful expression in these lines from *Child of the Salon*: "I feel that within me I concentrate unknown forces which emanate light, and that light will shine for me until my last breath of life. I feel that I am close to extracting from the abyss of my spirit a purpose which will become a source of happiness. For an hour, I was a saint. There was no passion or desire inside me — only sad thoughts, wistful sorrow, a melancholy which blesses the world — everything which lives, suffers, and errs."[1]

The new orphanage at 92 Krachmalna Street was dubbed the "Children's Home." The institute would embody Korczak's philosophy of childcare, which was that children had intrinsic value: they were people, not possessions, entitled to respect, nourishment, education, and vocational

---

[1]Quoted in "The Religious Consciousness of Janusz Korczak" by Krystyna Starczewska, *Dialogue and Universalism*, volume VII, no. 9–10, pg. 54, 1997. Published by the Institute of Philosophy, Warsaw University.

opportunity. Residents elected a parliament and served on a judicial council to hear complaints about their peers. They published a newspaper,
participated in small seminars on issues of the day, and presented plays to
which they would invite members of the community. Their classes
prepared them for work in the businesses of Warsaw or for further study at
university. Summers took them to camp in the countryside. Many of the
devoted staff, headed by Stefania Wilczynsk, who served as the chief exec-
utive officer, would remain with the orpha-nage throughout its thirty-year
history. They passionately shared the director's vision that orphans deserved
a loving environment. So radical was the Children's Home that children
advocates came from across Europe to serve internships in the new facility.

Conscription into the Czar's army again interrupted Korczak's life,
this time duty on the Eastern Front in World War I. In the war-
ravaged cities and countryside of the Ukraine, he observed that
children were the unlisted casualties when armies clashed. In these
hellish circumstances he assisted whenever possible in the care of desti-
tute children. He directed a shelter for Ukrainian children, organized
an orphanage in Kiev, and served as medical advisor for three other
orphanages, including a children's home established for Polish refugees.
He somehow found time and strength to compose a manual for childcare entitled *How to Love a Child*.

In the section of the book, "The Child in the Family," Korczak
wrote: "You say: 'My baby.' It is not. The child is a common property, he
belongs to the mother and father, the grandfathers and great-grand-
fathers. Some distant 'I' that was dormant in an army of forefathers, the
voice of a disintegrating, long forgotten coffin suddenly begins to
speak through your child."

Later he expounded:

"The entire present day upbringing is set on having an 'easy' child,
consistently, step by step, it strives to lull, squash, and destroy all that
goes into the making of the child's willpower and freedom, his back-
bone and the forcefulness of his demands and aims. 'Well-mannered,
obedient, good-natured and easy' with no thought given to the fact
that inside he will be will-less, and helpless in the affairs of life."[2]

[2]From *How to Love a Child*, in *Selected Works of Janusz Korczak*, translated by Jerzy Bachrach, published by the
National Science Foundation, Washington, D.C., 1967.

Korczak returned to Warsaw, now the capital of an independent nation, at war's end in 1918. The following year he contracted typhus while serving in a reserve unit of Poland's new army, while nursing him, his mother became ill with typhus and died. Korczak dealt with his grief by composing a series of prayers.

With military service and illness behind him, Korczak became a tireless crusader for children's rights. He lectured on childcare at Warsaw University. He defended children before the courts of the city. He founded a periodical for the writings of children. He accepted the directorship of a new orphanage for Catholic children. He would host a nationally broadcast radio program in which he assumed the persona of the "Old Doctor," dispensing advice for the proper love and care of children. He became Poland's Dr. Spock. His beloved Children's Home inspired widespread change in the way in which European countries viewed the treatment of disadvantaged children. Throughout his years of directorship of the Children's Home, Korczak maintained close daily supervision of its children.

Even with the press of such diverse duties, Korczak wrote copiously — articles and monographs dealing with educational philosophy, social reform, and childcare, and popular novels and stories.

King Matt the First

Published in 1923, Korczak's *King Matt the First* stands in the tradition of the *Bildungsroman*, a novel whose main subject is the moral, psychological, and intellectual development of a usually youthful main character. In addition to being a first-rate adventure story for young readers, *King Matt* offers valuable insight into the author's fundamental beliefs. Matt becomes king at age ten when his father dies. His kingdom is a landlocked European nation. Of pure heart, the boy-king strives to be a just leader. He is given wise counsel throughout his reign by an elderly doctor. The doctor guides the young monarch on a course of reconciliation among the peoples of his realm. Because the king has in disguise moved freely among the children of commoners, he knows firsthand of their needs and aspirations. The king strives to provide summer camps, free medicines, and equality before the law for his young subjects.

Disguised as a common foot-soldier, Matt learns of the futility of war in brutal battles fought in trenches. He survives the conspiracies of his adult cabinet ministers, who are solely driven by a thirst for power. When the king becomes vengeful or impulsive, the old doctor steers him back toward diplomatic engagement with his adversaries. From his counselor-physician, Matt learns patience and forbearance as each of his reforms are opposed.

Using gold procured on a journey to an African kingdom, Matt establishes two parliaments, one for adults, the other for children. He convenes an international conference of kings in an effort to promote peace and international cooperation. Against a backdrop of factional fighting, the children propose a series of reforms. When adults and children briefly trade places and responsibilities, civil disorder threatens the nation.

The children of the kingdom adopt as their symbol a green flag.

Neighboring countries conspire with traitors in Matt's own country to defeat his army. Captured, tried, and convicted before a tribunal of victorious generals, Matt, in golden chains, is led through the capital. He seems oblivious to crowds of detractors and supporters. Dry-eyed, he contemplates the blue sky and seems intent on other, more enduring matters. The final march of the young king would find an eerie parallel in the final days of Janusz Korczak.

Matt is led through the city:

> He walked down the middle of the street, still bound in golden chains. The streets were lined with soldiers, and behind them the people of the capital.
>
> It was a beautiful day. The sun was shining. Everyone had come out to see their king one last time. Many people had tears in their eyes. But Matt did not see these tears, though that would have made it easier for him to go to his death.
>
> Those who loved Matt said not a word, because they were afraid to express their love and respect for him in the presence of the enemy. Besides, what could they shout? They were used to shouting "Long live the King!" But how could they shout now, when the king was going to his death?"[3]

---

[3]*King Matt the First.* Translated by Richard Lourie. New York, Farrar, Straus and Giroux, 1986.

The doctor presented a personal message to each child who completed his or her stay in the Children's Home:

We did not give you God, because you must look and find Him within yourself.

We did not give you love of country, because your heart and reason must dictate your own choice.

We did not give you love of Man, because love comes from forgiveness which must be discovered through effort.

We did give you one thing — a longing for a better life, a life of truth and justice which you must build for yourself.

We hope that this longing will lead you to God, to country, and to love."[4]

In the 1930s a rising tide of anti-Semitism in Poland led to Korczak's dismissal from the directorship of the Catholic orphanage. His radio program was cancelled. He visited Palestine to consider relocation of his orphanage. His ties to his native land proved too strong, however, and he returned to Warsaw dedicated to the maintenance of his beloved orphanage in that city.

The beginning of the end for Korczak, the staff and children of the orphanage, and indeed for all of the Jews of Poland began on September 1, 1939 with the invasion of the country by German forces. In mid-month, Russia invaded from the east. Within a week, the German army surrounded Warsaw, the capital city. By month's end, following continuous, devastating bombardment, Warsaw surrendered. The Jews of the city now faced extermination at the hands of the Nazis.

The campaign to isolate and eventually to kill the Jews began at once. Jews were excluded from food lines. Their dwellings were ransacked and their belongings confiscated. Each Jew had to wear an identifying yellow star at all times. Jews were pressed into forced labor battalions. Random violence and summary executions were commonplace. In Warsaw, as in other Polish cities, Nazis appointed Jewish leaders to a council, or

---

[4]Quoted in the preface by Martin Wolins to *Selected Works of Janusz Korczak, op. cit.*

Judenrat, to carry out their edicts. Despite the best efforts of members of the Warsaw *Judenrat* to ameliorate living conditions, the relentless program of brutality toward Jews did not abate.

Within months of their victory, the Nazis established the first Jewish ghetto in the town of Lodz. The ghetto would allow easier control over Jews and other undesirables, such as Gypsies. Once concentrated within a ghetto, the captive population could more readily be deported to labor or death camps. While the Jews of Warsaw had been progressively segregated within their city, the formal announcement of their relocation within a walled ghetto did not come until October 12, 1940, which, in a cruel and deliberate twist, was Yom Kippur. In mid-November Nazi authorities sealed the Ghetto.

Henceforth, any passage to and from the Ghetto was strictly regulated at fortified gates. Four hundred thousand Jews, almost a third of the pre-war population of Warsaw, were crammed into an area of approximately one square mile. Gypsies and Jews from other areas of Poland were now relocated there. Starvation, disease, exposure, and the random brutality of Nazi authorities claimed 5000 to 6000 lives each month. Forced labor brigades were marched from the city, never to be heard from again.

★   ★   ★

I find the many historical accounts of the Warsaw Ghetto overwhelming. I found more emotionally manageable contact with the time of such horror in the photographic archives of the Holocaust Memorial Museum and in two movies, one simply entitled *Korczak,* the other *The Third Reich, In Color (Das dritte Reich – in Farbe).* The archives contrast photographs of pre-World War II Jewish life in Poland with harrowing images captured by German photographers in the Ghetto.

Two photographs especially haunt me. A picture of 1930 shows dark-haired 9-year-old Dorka Solnitski in a formal pose in the Children's Home. Clad in a black ruffled dress, black stockings, and lace-up leather shoes, she stands next to an upholstered chair, one arm resting atop its back, the other resting upon an arm of the chair. She looks resolutely at the camera. This child means business. She will attend the University, and once she has met the qualifications of a teacher she will join the staff at the Children's Home, where she will spend the rest of her life.

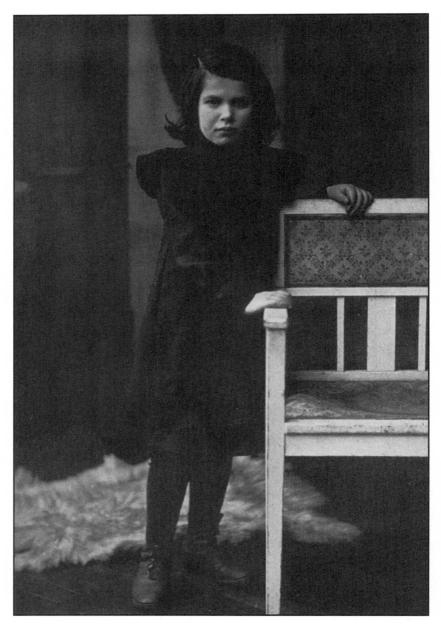

Dorka Solnitski at 9 years old, resident, later teacher, at the Children's Home.
(Photograph courtesy of Beit Lohamei Haghetaot –
The Ghetto Fighters' House, Western Galilee, Israel.)

A second photograph shows an emaciated child of similar age. Her black hair is curly, and she too wears a black dress. She is seated, her back against the bullet-pocked facade of a building. She looks askance from the camera; her dark-circled eyes have no luster. They seem to focus upon something in the distance. Her left hand rests beneath her younger sister who is stretched across her lap. Her right hand rests upon the dying girl's chest. A filthy coat covers the thin form of the younger girl who is unconscious and close to death. Her thinning hair suggests severe vitamin deficiency. Possibly she has typhus, a scourge in the packed streets of the Ghetto. I presume they are orphans. What will the older girl do with her sister's corpse? Will the younger sister find some slight comfort before she dies?

Korczak (1990) seamlessly intersperses dramatized segments with contemporary German newsreels of the Ghetto. The movie had limited distribution in the United States. When I saw *Korczak* in a Philadelphia cinema, the audience sat in stunned silence at the end of the movie before rising in unison to applaud. The tribute, I suspect, was directed as much to Janusz Korczak, his staff, and their children as to the actors, director, and producers of the movie.

The Third Reich, In Color (1998) includes footage of the fall of Poland and the Warsaw Ghetto. Evil is given a human face in this selection of movies by Hitler's personal photographer. The camera captures Hitler and his inner circle of advisors at play, at patriotic rallies, and at the executions of opponents. The camera almost casually records the faces of the starved, brutalized Jews of Warsaw.

★   ★   ★

When the order arrived to move to the Ghetto, Korczak, his staff, and the children had little time to pack their provisions and belongings. Leaving their home at in Krachmalna Street, they traveled in horse-drawn wagons to cramped quarters in a former school building. At the gate to the Ghetto, Nazi soldiers hijacked a wagonload of precious potatoes. When Korczak appeared before the Nazi authorities the following day to protest the theft, he was beaten and thrown into prison. But for the intervention of wealthy friends who raised a ransom, he probably would have died in captivity.

Until the very end the orphanage sustained its traditions of classes, seminars, and adherence to its democratic traditions. Korczak and his staff begged and cajoled for food and fuel to sustain the shrinking population of children. In October 1941, the Nazis contracted the ghetto by one-third. With scant notice the doctor, his staff, and their children had to move again, this time to even smaller quarters in a former merchants' club. A small house next door would house the staff.

Soon Korczak assumed the further responsibility of directing a broken and demoralized public orphanage of one thousand children. This facility would be little more than a place for abandoned or orphaned children to die.

Janusz Korczak kept a diary intermittently during his time in the Ghetto. In this remarkable memoir, found and placed in safekeeping after the final eviction of the orphans from their home, Korczak mixed auto-biographical fragments with clinical observations of his children and musings of his fundamental beliefs in the rights of children. Reading this powerful work, I sense Korczak struggling to hold on to his life for the sake of the guidance and strength that only he can give to his children.

In a lengthy entry of May 29, 1942 he writes:

How quickly the hours pass. Just now it was midnight — and already it's three in the morning. I had a visitor in my bed.

Mendelek had a bad dream. I carried him to my bed. He stroked my face (!) and went to sleep.

He squeals. He's uncomfortable.

"Are you asleep?"

He stares surprised with his black monkeylike beads of eyes.

"You were in the dormitory. Do you want to go back to your own bed?"

"Am I in your way?"

"Lie down at the other end. I'll bring you the pillow."

"Fine."

"I'll be writing. If you're frightened, come back."

"O.K."[5]

[5]Korczak, Janusz. *Ghetto Diary.* New York, Holocaust Library, 1978.

Amid the daily horrors of the Ghetto the children rehearsed for their final play, *The Post Office* by Rabindranath Tagore. Typed tickets were distributed to friends and supporters of the orphans:

Children's Care Unit.

We are not inclined if we are not sure.

We are sure that an hour of a beautiful tale of a thinker and a poet satisfies like a great feast.

Therefore we invite you to come on Saturday, July 18, 1942 at 4:30 P.M.

Dr. Korczak signed "Goldszmit" below his title, Director of the Orphans' Home.

A young friend of the Doctor added these lines:

From the unwritten review of the News:

The first real artistic spectacle since 1939!

More than a text — a mood!

More than a thrill — an experience!

More than actors — children!

No admission charge.[6]

The Post Office

Rabindranath Tagore, at the time widely considered the greatest writer in India, had won the 1913 Nobel Prize in Literature. The youngest of fourteen children of one of India's most renowned educators, Tagore spent his childhood years within the gloomy confines of the family home. Tagore wrote *The Post Office* in 1911, soon after the deaths of his wife, a son, and a daughter.

[6]Translation by Marzena Liruzej from a copy of a ticket in the U.S. Holocaust Memorial Museum Library.

The play opens with Amal, a young boy who is terminally ill, longing to leave the sickroom within his uncle's house. A doctor counsels that fresh air will surely kill the boy. He must remain confined. From his window Amal notices for the first time a magnificent new structure across the road. He learns that this will house a post office for the ruling Raja. The village watchman pauses at the window, humoring the lad with the promise that a Royal Physician will call upon Amal shortly to present him with a commission from the Raja to serve as a Royal Messenger. In this role Amal can traverse fields and forests and walk alongside streams. He will be free.

The florist's daughter stops at the window. She believes the story of the royal commission. She promises to bring Amal a fresh flower from the fields that he so longs to visit. A wanderer, disguised as a holy man, visits. He promises to Amal mantras which will remove all barriers to travel into the wild beauty of nature.

A prankster, stating that he bears a letter from the Raja, presents Amal with a blank piece of paper. No longer able to read, the boy gives the paper to the wanderer who improvises a message that the Raja will soon visit.

To the astonishment of all, the Royal Herald appears followed by the Royal Physician:

Raja's physician: What's this? All closed up?! Open up, open up, open all the doors and windows. How are you feeling young fellow?

Amal: Quite well, very well, Doctor. My illness is gone, my pain is gone. Now everything is open — I can see the stars, shining on the far side of darkness.

Physician: When the Raja comes in the dead of night, will you rise and go forth with him?

Amal: I will, I have the will. I long to go forth. I will ask the Raja to show me the Pole Star in the heavens. Perhaps I have seen it many times, and have not recognized it.

Physician: The Raja will show you all things. (To Uncle) Please make the room clean and decorate it with flowers to greet our Raja . . . .

Now you must all be calm. It is coming, coming, his sleep is coming. I will sit beside his pillow as he drifts off. Blow out the lamp, let the starlight come in, his sleep has arrived.[7]

The florist's daughter returns with a flower for Amal's pillow. She asks of the Royal Physician when Amal will awaken. She is assured that Amal will arise when the Raja arrives. Then Amal will be summoned into service as a Royal Messenger.

★　　★　　★

Freedom to roam awaits the virtuous child who patiently and optimistically endures illness and suffering. The lesson cannot have been lost on the orphans who attended the performance.

Korczak's diary entry of July 18 describes the reception of the play:

The next day, that was yesterday — the play. *The Post Office* by Tagore. Applause, handshakes, smiles, efforts at cordial conversation. (The chairwoman looked over the house after the performance and pronounced that though we are cramped, that genius Korczak had demonstrated that he could work miracles even in a rat hole.)

This is why others have been allotted palaces.

I could find no mention of Tagore or *The Post Office* in earlier writings of Korczak. Possibly, the death of Tagore in August 1941 stimulated Korczak's recollection of a cherished dramatic work. The play insists that every virtuous child will be rewarded with an eternal life of freedom. Korczak's diary shows that he harbored no delusions that his children would survive. *The Post Office* demonstrated poignantly for the children who filled the roles and composed much of the audience that their present travails would precede a life of freedom in beautiful, natural surroundings—the antithesis of the stifling, deadly Ghetto.

Presentation of this play was risky because the Nazis had placed Tagore's works on their list of banned literary works. If the Nazis had learned of the performance of *The Post Office,* this may account for their

---

[7] *The Post Office.* Translated by Krishna Dutta and Andrew Robinson. In *Rabindranath Tagore: An Anthology.* St. Martin's Press, New York, 1997.

seizure, several days after the performance, of Estreka Winogron, friend and assistant of Korczak and director of the performance of the play.

Three days later Korczak wrote in his diary on the eve of his birthday:

Tomorrow I shall be sixty-three or sixty-four years old. For some years, my father failed to obtain my birth certificate. I suffered a few difficult moments over that. Mother called it gross negligence: being a lawyer, father should not have delayed in the matter of the birth certificate . . .

It is a difficult thing to be born and to learn to live. Ahead of me is a much easier task: to die. After death, it may be difficult again, but I am not bothering about that. The last year, month or hour.

I should like to die consciously, in possession of my faculties. I don't know what I should say to the children by way of farewell. I should want to make clear to them only this — that the road is theirs to choose, freely.

The Final March

Janusz Korczak made the final entry in his diary on August 4, 1942:

I am watering the flowers, the poor orphanage plants, the plants of the Jewish orphanage. The parched soil breathed with relief.

A guard watched me as I worked. Does that peaceful work of mine at six o'clock in the morning annoy him or move him? He stands looking on, his legs wide apart . . .

I am watering the flowers. My bald head in the window. What a splendid target.

He has a rifle. Why is he standing and looking on calmly?

He has no orders to shoot.

And perhaps he was a village teacher in civilian life, or a notary, a street sweeper in Leipzig, a waiter in Cologne?

What would he do if I nodded to him? Waved my hand in a friendly gesture?

Perhaps he doesn't even know that things are — as they are?

He may have arrived only yesterday, from far away.

★   ★   ★

Two days later, Nazi soldiers surrounded the orphanage and ordered its evacuation. Large-scale seizures of Ghetto residents had occurred sporadically for weeks. Guards marched their captives to the rail depot, the *Umschlagplatz*, where they were forced aboard boxcars that would take them to the death camp at Treblinka. Now the German authorities determined that the Ghetto would be cleared of all institutionalized children.

Upon receiving the order to leave the orphanage, Korczak and the ten surviving members of his staff assembled the children, making sure that each had provisions for a journey. A photograph purportedly from that fateful morning shows Korczak and the children. He wears a black overcoat. The boys and girls wear jackets and cloth backpacks. A female staff member, possibly Dorka Solnitski, assists.

Their march on that hot August day takes them the length of the Ghetto to the *Umschlagplatz*. They wait quietly at the train station in the midst of pandemonium. At a signal from the Doctor, the children and their guardians board the boxcars that will take them to their awful deaths.

The Warsaw Ghetto Uprising would begin in April 1943 and last a month. Of the 56,000 Jews captured, about 30,000 were either immediately shot or transported to death camps. The remainder were sent to labor camps. As Himmler had ordered, the Ghetto was razed to the ground.

A Visit to Poland: November 2000

From the moment that I completed Ms. Lifton's biography of Korczak, I knew that I would some day have to visit Warsaw and Treblinka. That opportunity presented itself in November 2000. I would have three days for my visit. I had studied maps and reviewed my books of Ghetto history for weeks before my journey.

157

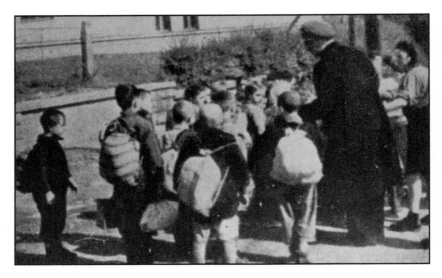

*Purported photograph of Janusz Korczak and his children in the Warsaw Ghetto
shortly before transportation to Treblinka.
(Courtesy of Yad Vashem Photo Archives, USHMM Photo Archives.)*

My hotel lay close upon Sienna Street at the southern end of the former Ghetto. My requests of the concierge for information or maps relating to the Ghetto induced blank stares. Through the wonderful assistance of Marzena Lizurej, a Polish friend in New York, I met my guide, Barbara Kandora, a young school teacher from Southern Poland. I would see the Ghetto with her help.

Apart from a brief break for coffee and cake, Barbara and I walked from noon until six. We sought fragments of the Ghetto's encircling wall. The first abutted a dark, crumbling tenement, one of the few structures left partially standing after the Ghetto was razed in the spring of 1943. The wall joined the ground floor of the tenement that had itself formed part of the Ghetto perimeter.

With difficulty we located the surviving gateway through which the Nazis controlled entry and egress from the Ghetto. The tattered archway gave no hint of its previous, sinister use.

We walked to Pawiak Prison, the dreaded death-house where Korczak had been imprisoned for protesting the theft of the orphanage's potatoes. Obituary notices of Poles who had died in the prison covered the trunk of a twisted dead tree that stood before the low bunker. Candles burned at its base.

We walked the Path of Remembrance whose granite blocks commemorate various individuals, events, and places connected with the Ghetto. At the end of the Path, we reached the *Umschlagplatz*, the site of the railroad siding where Jews were loaded into boxcars bound for Treblinka. But for a German tour group who paused briefly at the memorial, we were its only visitors. The simple, marble structure opened on its east end to parallel marble tracks marking the course of the rails upon which the death-trains began their journeys. Images of shattered tree trunks adorned the iron arc over the entrance. The names of some of the families deported from the station were etched into the walls of the interior. I could feel the scene of the orphans' departure.

As light faded on that November evening, we sought our final goal, an orphanage constructed upon the site of Dr. Korczak's original building at 92 Krachmalna Street. Our maps were contradictory. Street names had been altered first by German forces, then by Poland's Communist government. My guide sought directions to no avail from passers-by and shop-owners. Barbara recalled having been shown the site on a visit with classmates to Warsaw years earlier.

Grayish-yellow light suffused the narrow street. Two men struggled to disarm the burglar alarm on a battered Fiat parked before a dilapidated repair shop. Cars and vans lined both sides of the street. Over the top of the last of these I could see a cream-colored building. A few steps further and we stood before a four-story structure which bore a stunning resemblance to the photographs I had seen of Korczak's orphanage. We entered the courtyard over which presided a large bust of the Doctor. A groundskeeper affirmed that the building served as an orphanage. He did not know of the ethnic or religious composition of its residents. Yes, we could enter, but we should not disturb the staff or the students. Plaques on the front wall commemorated Korczak, his staff, and the earlier Jewish orphans.

A short hallway led us into an auditorium, a raised stage at one end, faded photographs of the original orphanage along the walls. The floor plan had remained loyal to the initial building on that site. I knew that I was on sacred territory. I paused and offered a silent prayer for all the orphans and their caregivers who had shared this place. My guide dabbed at tears. From upstairs came scratchy notes of a classical record. We could hear muffled voices of children from a dining hall. It was time to close our first day.

Treblinka proved a greater challenge. Officials of Poland's offices of tourism seemingly do not wish to facilitate visits to the site. We began our journey at nine in the morning aboard an ancient train from Warsaw's Central Station. Our destination was Malkinia, the railhead closest to Treblinka. By halfway, our second-class compartment was jammed with passengers and their large boxes and suitcases. The single toilet that served the car no longer functioned.

A ninety-minute journey brought us to the deserted concrete bunker that constituted Malkinia Station. Barbara negotiated expertly with a taxi driver to take us the fourteen kilometers to Treblinka. He agreed to wait and then return us to the train station. The fare arranged by Barbara was far less than that initially sought by the driver.

We passed through the village of Treblinka, six kilometers removed from the camp. We came to a narrow single lane bridge over a river. The right-of-way served both auto and train. A traffic light signaled when it was safe for cars to proceed over the shared bridge. A nearby bridge for cars still lay in ruins from bombardment over half a century ago.

A modest, faded sign marked the turnoff to the camp. The narrow blacktop ended at a concrete shell. An empty military ambulance was the only other vehicle parked at the memorial. Signs had rusted, and several had fallen. We located a footpath that took us to a rail-bed marked by concrete crossties, perhaps a foot tall. A spur ended alongside the outlines of a platform.

At the platform new arrivals were separated by sex and directed into barracks where they were ordered to remove their clothing and submit to clipping of their hair and beards. The prisoners were then directed along "the road to heaven," a path lined by whip-wielding guards, that led to the gas chamber. Slave laborers removed the bodies and stacked them in ditches; later, to eradicate all traces of these crimes, the wholesale burning of corpses began. At its peak, Treblinka could in a single day "process" 12,000 to 14,000 people.

Another path led to a crematorium now marked by twin stone

pillars upon whose capstone are chiseled hands and faces in expressions of anguish. Alongside the path to the memorial stood stone monuments commemorating the nations whose captive citizens had been sent to Treblinka — Greece, Poland, USSR, Estonia, Czechoslovakia, Hungary, and Germany.

The memorial sat in a field of irregular grey stones, each two to three feet high, each inscribed with the name of a village or town from which victims had been sent to die in this camp of hell. I searched for a special memorial described by Ms. Lifton. I found it close to the central monument, a larger, white stone inscribed "Janusz Korczak, Henryk Goldszmit, and the Children." A nearby rectangular slab declared, "Nigdj Wiecej" — "Never Again." Perhaps a million people were murdered at this site.

Treblinka was the only Nazi death camp to experience a full-scale revolt. On August 2, 1943, guards were attacked and buildings set ablaze. About 300 inmates escaped into the forest; about 100 survived the massive Nazi manhunt.

Emotionally exhausted by our visit, Barbara and I returned to the empty train station at Malkinia. The ticket agent in Warsaw had been unable or unwilling to sell us a roundtrip ticket. No one manned the office at Malkinia. We were among six passengers who flagged the 1430 train. We assumed that we could purchase tickets for Warsaw once we were on board. Hardly had we taken our seats on rickety orange plastic seats, than we were accosted by a red-faced, foul-tempered conductor. I had witnessed him taking money for tickets from other passengers. The fact that I spoke no Polish and had an American passport set him off. He berated my guide and threatened to have us thrown off the train. Ever the pessimist, I foresaw at least a night in custody at some remote town. A model of calm, Barbara instructed me to sit tight while she conversed animatedly with the conductor. We were allowed to remain aboard after paying a fifty-zloty fine. From the expressions on the faces of the other passengers, I sensed the residuum of fear and anger that persisted from years of arbitrary rule in Poland.

Our train broke down twenty kilometers outside Warsaw, but a relief train brought us to the eastern side of the city. A series of bus rides brought us to the Central Station where I bade farewell to my ever-patient guide. I believe that she was on a personal mission of sorts during our shared travel. The Ghetto, the orphanage, and Treblinka had moved her deeply. I sensed that she was filling in blanks of a history lesson that had been taught to her in school. I wondered how those lessons matched what we had seen together.

On my final day in Warsaw I had three visits to make. The first was the Museum of Jewish History. I had anticipated seeing an exhibit on the life of Janusz Korczak. For reasons I could never discern, that exhibit had been dismantled days earlier before its announced date of closure. The museum's permanent exhibit of the Ghetto was, however, informative and poignant.

My second goal was the Jewish Cemetery, closed when Barbara and I had first tried to visit. Shards from headstones smashed by Nazi occupiers were set in the stucco of a wall that led to a statue of Korczak and his children. This is their symbolic burial site. The black monument portrays Korczak on the final march. He carries a young child while holding the hand of another. Four other children cluster to their rear. The monument is in severe disrepair. Wire mesh can be seen in scattered gaps in the black plaster. I wonder how much longer the memorial can endure. My enquiries to Polish officials regarding the rehabilitation of the statue have never been answered. Nearby a segment of Ghetto wall had been relocated. A teddy bear and inlaid photo-graphs of children rested at the base along with several lighted candles.

Finally, I located in a guide to Holocaust sites a segment of wall within a courtyard at 55 Sienna Street, the Children's Home final address, reached with great difficulty because of the moat-like barriers presented by two thoroughfares. A pocked concrete archway led into an overgrown courtyard surrounded on three sides by office and apartment buildings. To the left stood a thirty-foot-long brick fragment of original wall from the larger Ghetto. Flowers, both planted and in bouquets, adorned the base of the structure. A small plaque in Polish was placed just beneath a two-brick gap in the wall. Adjacent to it, a smaller bronze plaque noted in English that the two bricks had been removed to the Holocaust Memorial Museum in Washington. A Polish lady approached the wall, bowed her head, and whispered a prayer. A photographer approached, offering in English to take her picture for a price. She uttered what I presume was a curse and gave him a universal sign of contempt with her gloved hand. She resumed her meditative posture before the wall.

I departed Warsaw later that day. Images and thoughts from my brief stay remain with me. My walk around the perimeter and through the former Ghetto made palpable in a way that books and photographs could not the horror of that chapter of the Holocaust. From the moment of invasion, the Nazis had intended to murder the Jews of Poland. The Nazis enlisted starvation and disease, stifling summertime heat and brutally cold winters, as their allies in this barbaric mission. I left Warsaw and Treblinka with a sense of proportion, of boundaries and distances. I could link specific events with the image of a street or a former entry gate. I could understand the physical stress of the forced walk of Korczak and the orphans to the train station. At the death camp modest distances separated arrival platform, changing stations, gas chambers, and crematorium. Perhaps uncertain at the moment of arrival as to their fates, the deportees to Treblinka would have no question as to what lay ahead once they felt the whips of the guards along the path to the gas chamber. The horrors are almost impossible to contemplate. I firmly believe that the orphans whom Korczak and his staff had so powerfully loved and taught marched to their deaths with an unshaken faith that they would awaken to freedom in the full beauties of nature.

Janusz Korczak had witnessed brutality before — in his nighttime rambles through the slums of Warsaw during his years of medical study and in his military service in the Russian army. He had survived near-suicidal depression upon the death of his mother. He conceptualized an alternative universe, an ideal world in which all children would have respect, love, and protection before the law. Children in turn could point adults to the same possibilities for their lives.

At the conclusion of the movie *Koczak,* the train bound for Treblinka stops in mid-journey. The door opens, and Korczak and his children joyfully bound into the surrounding fields in the same fashion that Amal dreamed in *The Post Office.* This was the journey of the spirit for which the Doctor prepared his charges.

My visit to Poland was finally a pilgrimage to honor a personal hero and a universal saint. His teachings are timeless. His courageous example of compassion for the poorest and weakest of society begs for emulation in our conflicted world.

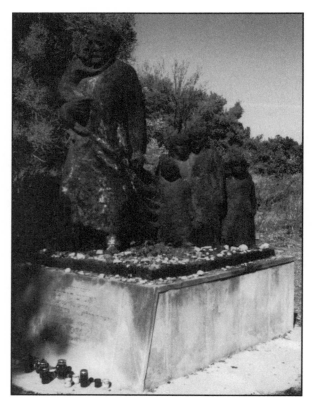

The Janusz Korczak Memorial in Warsaw.

SOURCES AND ACKNOWLEDGMENTS

The King of Children: A Biography of Janusz Korczak by Betty Jean Lifton (1988) merits inclusion in the personal libraries of physicians, advocates for child welfare, and indeed anyone who loves children. There are several English editions of Korczak's *Ghetto Diary,* an astonishing memoir written under heart-wrenching circumstances. Other works by Korczak in English are *King Matt the First,* featuring an introduction by Bruno Bettelheim (1986); *A Voice for the Child: The Inspirational Words of Janusz Korczak,* edited by Sandra Joseph (1999), and *When I Am Little Again and The Child's Right to Respect,* translated by E.P. Kulawiec (1992). A useful overview is provided in *Janusz Korczak: Universal Significance of His Work and Martyrdom (Dialogue and Universalism,* volume VII, numbers 9-10, Warsaw University, 1997). In 1990 *Korczak,* a movie in Polish with English subtitles, appeared in limited release. New Yorker Films has released the movie in VHS format. Beautifully acted, this movie deserves inclusion in the libraries of medical schools.

For the great Indian author, see Krishna Dutta and Andrew Robinson's *Rabindranath Tagore: The Myriad-Minded Man* (1995). A translation of *The Post Office* appears in their *Rabindranath Tagore: An Anthology* (1997). For information on the Holocaust and the Warsaw Ghetto in particular, I have relied upon a number of books: *The War Against the Jews* by Lucy Dawidowicz (1975); *Forgotten Holocaust: The Poles under German Occupation, 1939-1944* by Richard Lukas (1986); *The Jews of Warsaw, 1939-1943: Ghetto, Underground, Revolt* by Israel Gutman (1989); *The Bravest Battle: The 28 Days of the Warsaw Ghetto Uprising* by Dan Kurzman (1993); *Words to Outlive Us: Eyewitness Accounts from the Warsaw Ghetto* edited by Michal Grynberg (2002); *The Destruction of the European Jews* by Raul Hilberg (1967); *The Warsaw Diary of Adam Czerniakow* edited by Raul Hilberg, Stanislaw Staron, and Josef Kermisz (1979); and *Treblinka* by Jean-François Steiner (1967).

The generous and patient staff of the United States Holocaust Memorial Museum Library guided me through that institution's extensive photograph collection and literary resources. These visits were crucial to my understanding of the Holocaust generally and Janusz Korczak in particular.

EPILOGUE

AN ANATOMY OF COURAGE

—∾∾∾—

If we are fortunate, and the majority of us are, we are born and grow up normally. We arrive with the parts and enzymatic systems that ensure reasonable function of our bodies as we grow from infancy. A variety of caregivers, including parents, grandparents, older siblings, and teachers, will nurture us physically, spiritually, and intellectually until we are sufficiently mature to undertake choices of our own. Yet there is no magical, set age at which maturity can be presumed. Indeed, maturity may well be a lifelong process rather than a particular landmark in our lives.

The ordinary people whom I have described made under a variety of challenging circumstances choices that are rightly termed "courageous" or "heroic" in that they exceeded what we would expect of most people faced with similar dilemmas. Because of their overuse in the popular media, however, the terms "courageous" and "heroic" bear closer examination. Courage exhibited in an athletic competition is certainly different from courage displayed in the rescue of a child in danger.

Courage or fortitude, along with prudence, temperance, and justice, is one of the four cardinal virtues upheld as primary foundations of moral character by ancient and medieval thinkers. The third edition of the *American Heritage Dictionary of the English Language* describes *kerd* as the Indo-European root of "courage." *Kerd* means "heart." As the word wandered through Latin it became *cor* before evolving into *corage* in Middle English.

"Hero" derives from the Indo-European root *ser-*, "to protect." *Heros,* "protector," became its Greek and Latin form. In Greek mythology heroes were men who exhibited great courage and enjoyed the favor of the gods. I have used the term "hero" in this book to denote men *and* women who have exhibited courage.

To understand courage as a moral trait I turned to a variety of sources. In Book III of *The Nicomachean Ethics,* Aristotle contends that moral purpose is more closely related to virtue and is a better criterion of character than actions themselves are:

It is clear that moral purpose is something voluntary. (Chapter IV)

In Chapter IX, Aristotle describes the courageous person:

Strictly speaking, then, we may call a person courageous if he is fearless in facing a noble death, and in all such sudden emergencies as bring death near, and therefore especially in facing the chances of war.

Finally, in Chapter XI, Aristotle defines courage:

Courage then . . . is a mean state in regard to the causes of confidence and fear, in such circumstances as have been described; and it chooses action or endures pain because this is the noble course or because the opposite course is disgraceful.

My thinking about courage has been helped considerably by André Comte-Sponville's *Small Treatise on the Great Virtues.* He writes:

That which we respect about courage, then, and which has its culmination in self-sacrifice is first of all the acceptance or incurring of risk without selfish motivation; in other words, a form, if not always of altruism, then at least of disinterestedness, detachment, or a distancing from the self. That, in any case, is what we find in courage that is morally worthy of respect. (pp 47, 49).

Comte-Sponville elaborates on the moral anchoring of courage:

> [C]ourage as a virtue always presupposes some form of selflessness, altruism, or generosity. Virtuous courage certainly does not rule out a certain insensitivity to fear or even a certain relish for it. But it does not presuppose them. This kind of courage is not absence of fear but the capacity to overcome it by a stronger and more generous will. It is no longer (or no longer just) physiology: it is fortitude, moral strength in the face of danger. It is no longer a passion: it is a virtue, one that is the precondition of all the others. It is no longer the courage of the tough: it is the courage of the gentle, and of heroes.

Jonathan Lear in *Happiness, Death, and the Remainder of Life* uses texts from Aristotle and Freud in addressing Man's search for a purposeful life. He too writes of courage:

> The only way into the courageous life is via habituation, beginning in childhood, in performing courageous acts. If all goes well, such a person will develop a stable psychic condition in which he can both judge well, in any given set of circumstances, the courageous thing to do, and, in making that judgment, be so motivated to act . . . Now there are two features of an ethical virtue, like courage, which are inherently linked, though they may seem to tilt in opposite directions. Every ethical virtue is a source of creativity and an occasion for repetition. First, creativity: no matter how varied experience is, no matter what strange peculiarities a person may be faced with, the courageous person will be sensitive to what in those circumstances is the courageous thing to do . . . courage is also a form of repetition. For a courageous person, every set of circumstances and every action are implicitly or explicitly brought back to the question: what, in this set of circumstances, is the courageous thing to do? (pp 63-4).

Thus informed by Aristotle, Comte-Sponville, and Lear, I comprehend courage as a voluntary or learned virtue that directs its possessor, or hero, to face danger in whatever form in a spirit of altruism. Danger may be manifest as a threat of death, injury, or disgrace; danger may take the form of ignorance, injustice, or brutality. Courage is not reckless, nor is it prideful, nor cruel.

The heroes of my early years seemed to have qualities of strength and self-assuredness that elevated them to a distinct category of personhood. While we could revere such individuals and try to emulate their behavior, we had little hope of ever attaining their status. Subsequent years have proved the fallacy of this conception. I realize that we are surrounded by heroes, most of whose actions are often unnoticed, and that we are all potential heroes-in-waiting. I further realize that oftentimes heroism is not manifest simply in one great action but in a series of interconnected actions over many years or an entire lifetime. The heroes that I have described in the preceding chapters illustrate this and reflect the various facets of courageous or heroic behavior.

Corydon Wassell, Billie Dyer, and Vera Palmer exemplify the heroism of healers in times of warfare. Against a disorienting backdrop of sophisticated weaponry and mass casualties, they exhibited a tireless devotion to their patients. Each of the three, while often caring for large numbers of patients, never ignored the particular needs of the individual. Doctor Wassell spent time during his daily rounds at the bedside of each sailor, listening and reassuring. He recognized that a cigarette, a cold beer, or a serving of ice cream had a role in healing his patients. Doctor Dyer could sympathize with the mothers of downed enemy pilots. Nurse Palmer could give hope to a G.I. who had lost his feet to frostbite.

These three healers also exemplify courage as a collaborative or catalytic endeavor. Each, through their examples, lifted spirits and nurtured courage among their patients. The sailors under Dr. Wassell's care rolled bandages, evacuated bedfast buddies to safety, and even moved into the burn unit to assist in the care of shipmates with severer injuries. Doctor Dyer worked to convert even the most dilapidated, barren facility into a clean and efficient center for care for his patients. Nurse Palmer brought an inexhaustible sense of calm and hope to a shock tent ever on the verge of collapse before the pressure of waves of casualties.

Billie Dyer and Lonnie Boaz had to surmount enduring barriers of racism in providing care for their patients. The former was but a generation removed from slavery; the latter lost his father to a hate crime. Neither doctor succumbed to anger or bitterness despite insults and segregation. Each physician kept before him the goal of providing the best possible health care. At the same time, both were examplars of equanimity under pressure who gave heart — or courage — to other African Americans.

Like Drs. Wassell, Dyer, and Boaz and Nurse Palmer, Dr. Woodrow Dodson exemplified devotion and compassion. In his lifelong commitment to the citizens of Canton, Missouri, he brought persistence and steadiness to a career of sixty years. Often he worked alone. His devotion demanded daily study of medical journals and his Bible so that he would be factually and spiritually ready for the next day's demands. He postponed relaxation and sacrificed time with his family to meet the needs of his patients, each of whom he considered a friend.

Paulette McGill and Barry Walker manifested courage in several ways. They lived with the uncertainties of chronic illness and recurring episodes of intense pain. They accepted the likelihood that their lives would end prematurely. They shared a devotion to teach and to comfort others. Paulette felt beloved within her family and sought to convey this love to her young students. She regularly brought music performed on piano, organ, and violin to her students and to members of her church community so that they might find in that medium a serenity such as she enjoyed. Barry sought in every contact to raise the level of cheer. A comforter by nature, he carefully instructed his family and legions of friends in how to approach death. He forbade mourning, insisting that life called for celebration and mutual support. Paulette and Barry always sought to avoid alarming or upsetting their families and friends. They bore pain quietly and resolutely.

Hat Chau refused to be dehumanized. He withstood years of the most heinous treatment imaginable, sustaining a vision of what life could be. He took, in effect, a lonely stand on behalf of all of us, insisting that beauty always lay at the horizon of human experience. His father and mother and his special mentor, Charlotte Harris, taught him and gave him strength during his perilous journey to manhood. Hat presents us with orchids to give us pause to contemplate the loveliness inherent in life.

Sometimes courage boils down to a continuing commitment simply to go forward. My unnamed friend at summer camp could not lay down a painful, emotional burden that cast a long shadow over her life but, in much the same way as Hat Chau in the slave labor camp, she refused to give in to despair. I do not know if she had a larger vision of possibilities that gave strength to her or if she devoted herself to getting through one day at a time. She built a family life and, I think, prevented the chaos of child abuse from spilling into later generations.

Norman Maclean represents a special example of intellectual courage. He visited the site of the tragedy at Mann Gulch while the ashes were still warm. He was troubled by the loss of so many young lives. He suspected that blame for the tragedy had been wrongly assigned. At a time in life when most persons would be content to compile memoirs or relax on a porch, he made repeated, exhausting treks into the canyon and compiled data from multiple sources to explain the disaster. He could not tolerate false assumptions being given the credence of fact, especially if this impugned the integrity of the leader of the smokejumper team. The dedication of Norman Maclean to arrive at the truth demonstrates that retirement never frees us from similar obligations.

Janusz Korczak is the complete avatar of courage. Early in his life he identified a major societal illness — the abuse in Polish society of poor and orphaned children. He analyzed its causes and dedicated his life to its correction. He recruited dedicated associates who would work with him and the children until their murders at Treblinka. In addition to his daily work in his orphanage as physician and teacher, he tirelessly advocated a better life for all children through lectures, radio broadcasts, writings, and appearances in court. His life exemplifies integrity, hope, love, and courage. When offered chances to escape the Ghetto, he elected to remain with his children to teach them a final lesson of how to remain strong and kind in the face of barbarity and death. Janusz Lorczak is a Hero for the Ages.

★   ★   ★

My heroes continue to sustain and inspire me.

WORKS CITED

Aristotle. *The Nicomachean Ethics.* J.E.C. Welldon, ed. and trans. Amherst, New York: Prometheus Books; 1987.

Comte-Sponville, André. *A Small Treatise on the Great Virtues: The Uses of Philosophy in Everyday Life.* Catherine Temerson, ed. and trans. New York; Metropolitan Books; 2001.

Lear, Jonathan. *Happiness, Death, and the Remainder of Life.* Cambridge, MA: Harvard University Press; 2000.

SELECTED READINGS
IN COURAGE

—⟨✦⟩—

Books continue to amaze, inform, and inspire me. I especially treasure five books that have given me insights into the complexities of courage.

In *The Diving Bell and the Butterfly* (1997), Jean-Dominique Bauby guides us into the world of the locked-in syndrome. Bauby, the editor of the French magazine *Elle,* had his world wrecked in December 1995 by a severe stroke that narrowed his ability to communicate to the blink of an eyelid. With the aid of devoted friends who would point to letters until a blink indicated his choice, Bauby composed a memoir during the next seven months. The "diving bell" of the title refers to his entrapment within his severely damaged body. The "butterfly" describes the freedom afforded to him by consciousness, memory, and imagination. Some of his caregivers appear brusque and impatient. Some of his friends stay away, uncertain how to conduct themselves in the presence of such trauma. Bauby dictated a monthly bulletin that was distributed to sixty friends:

> Thus was born a collective correspondence that keeps me in touch with those I love, and my hubris has had gratifying results. Apart from an irrecoverable few who maintain a stubborn silence, every-one now understands that he can join me in my diving bell, even if sometimes the diving bell takes me into unexplored territory. (pp 82-3)

A sunrise reflected upon a brick wall, visits with his children, subtle sounds that drift into his room—all are savored and described in stunning prose. After several months, however, Bauby senses quite accurately that the end is near:

> I am fading away. Slowly but surely. Like the sailor who watches the home shore gradually disappear, I watch my past recede. My old life still burns within me, but more of it is reduced to the ashes of memory. (p 77)

His memoir closes in August 1996:

> Does the cosmos contain keys for opening up my diving bell? A subway line with no terminus? A currency strong enough to buy my freedom back? We must keep looking. I'll be off now. (pp 131-2)

Jean-Dominique Bauby died two days before publication of his masterpiece of courage.

Poet and short-story writer Raymond Carver's last gift to us was *A New Path to the Waterfall*. Diagnosed with carcinoma of the lung in September 1987, Carver suffered metastases to his brain the following March and recurrences in his lungs three months later. In June 1988, Carver and his companion of eleven years, Tess Gallagher, married. He died in August of that year.

A New Path to the Waterfall, posthumously published in 1989, begins with a moving introductory essay by Ms. Gallagher. The volume contains 50 poems written during Carver's last few months. Like his better known short stories, Carver's poetry reflects his emotional honesty. The final poems show Carver's awareness of mortality while celebrating life. "Gravy" is one of them.

GRAVY

No other word will do. For that's what it was. Gravy.
Gravy, these past ten years.
Alive, sober, working, loving, and
being loved by a good woman. Eleven years
ago he was told he had six months to live
at the rate he was going. And he was going
nowhere but down. So he changed his ways
somehow. He quit drinking! And the rest?
After that it was *all* gravy, every minute
of it, up to and including when he was told about,
well, some things that were breaking down and
building up inside his head. "Don't weep for me,"
he said to his friends. "I'm a lucky man.
I've had ten years longer than I or anyone
expected. Pure gravy. And don't forget it." (p 118)

I had never heard of the French novelist Alphonse Daudet (1840-1897) until I read his notes on physical suffering, *Le Doulou* (*In the Land of Pain*). In addition to newly editing and translating the work (2002), British novelist Julian Barnes has provided a valuable introduction to Daudet and his times. Daudet suffered from tabes dorsalis, an end-stage of syphilis, that caused progressive loss of balance and bouts of shooting pain of almost unimaginable intensity. Morphine, visits to spas, and various medical treatments provided little relief. Twelve years would pass between Daudet's receiving this diagnosis and his death. Daudet kept notes and observations during the first nine years of this ordeal.

Varieties of pain.

Sometimes on the sole of the foot, an incision, a thin one, hair-thin. Or a penknife stabbing away beneath the big toenail. The torture of the boot. Rats gnawing at the toes with very sharp teeth.

And amid all these woes, the sense of a rocket climbing, climbing up into your skull, and then exploding as the climax of the show. (p 21)

Daudet struggled to maintain relationships with his family and friends. At spas and sanitaria to which he was referred, he eavesdropped and observed fellow patients with wit and sympathy.

> Painful hours spent at Julia's bedside (Mme. Daudet) . . . Fury at finding myself such a wreck, and too weak to nurse her. But my ability to feel sympathy and tenderness for others is still well alive, as is my capacity for emotional suffering, for emotional torment . . . And I'm glad of that, despite the terrible pains that returned today. (p 25)

In the Land of Pain takes us to Ground Zero of physical suffering. Pain repeatedly pressed Daudet to the limit of endurance. His intellect, artistry, and love of his wife allowed him to prevail.

In *The Railway Man* (1995), Eric Lomax presents a memoir of crushing brutality and ultimate forgiveness. A young radioman in the British army, Lomax was captured in the Japanese invasion of Singapore in early 1942. His captors transported him to Ban Pong in Thailand where he would work in the shops that supported the construction by POWs of the infamous Burma-Siam railroad that included the bridge over the River Kwai. When Lomax and several of his friends were found in possession of a homemade radio, they were subjected to days of torture and interrogation before being transported to prisons in Singapore. There he endured starvation and disease before being freed at war's end. He fought for decades to overcome the psycho-logical traumas of his imprisonment.

In 1989 Lomax learned that one of his Japanese interrogators, Nagase Takashi, survived. Nagase had been present during an episode of Lomax's water torture. Nagase had devoted his postwar years to atonement for his role in torturing POWs. Lomax initially planned to locate and to kill Nagase. A correspondence between his wife, Patti, and Nagase eventually led to a meeting of the one-time prisoner and his adversary at the site of the River Kwai bridge:

From about a hundred yards away I saw him walk out on to the bridge; he could not see me. It was important for me to have this last momentary advantage over him; it prepared me, even now that I no longer wanted to hurt him. I walked about a hundred yards to an open square, a kind of courtyard overlooking the river, where we had arranged to meet . . .

He began a formal bow, his face working and agitated, the small figure barely reaching my shoulder. I stepped forward, took his hand and said 'Ohayo gozaimasu, Nagase san, ogenki desu ka?' 'Good morning, Mr. Nagase, how are you?' (pp 262-3)

Lomax and Nagase and their wives visited the site of the railroad before traveling to Japan. The men forged a sympathy and an understanding that culminated in Lomax reading to Nagase a letter of forgiveness on their final day together.

Back in Thailand, at the Chungkai War Cemetary, when Patti and I walked off on our own, she had had a moment of doubt as she looked at the rows and rows of graves, and wondered whether we were doing the right thing after all. It was only a moment, for we both knew we had to be there. I said then: 'Sometime the hating has to stop.' (p 276)

Reynolds Price, master teacher, acclaimed novelist and short story writer, poet, and playwright presents in *A Whole New Life: An Illness and a Healing* (1994), a memoir of catastrophic illness, mind-tearing pain, disability, and ultimate return to the creative life. In 1984 a lymphoma was found in his spinal cord. Surgery and radiation destroyed the neoplasm but left Price paraplegic and in the grip of severe pain. His caregivers vary from indifferent to deeply empathetic. Two epiphanies occur in dreams, renewing for Price vital links to his religious faith. Gradually, he weaned himself from the narcotics prescribed for his pain. Friends and family members repeatedly rallied in support of him. He redesigned his home to accommodate his limitations. He resumed teaching and writing, professions that he pursues to this day.

I have heard him speak eloquently on National Public Radio of his new life.

> Was it disaster — all that time from my slapped-down sandal in spring '84 through the four years till I reentered life as a new contraption, inside and out? Is it still disaster, these ten years later? Numerous mouths and pairs of eyes have been, and still are, ready to tell me Yes every week. Very often occasional acquaintances will corner me on campus or at a party, then lean to my ear and ask how I am. When I tell them truthfully 'Fine,' their faces will crouch in solemn concern, and they'll say 'No, *really*. How *are* you?' I'll give them a skull-grin to cover my amusement at the common eagerness of so many otherwise decent souls to see a fellow creature buried. (p 178)

When I first read this memoir, I could handle only a few pages at a time, such is the intensity of Price's account of suffering. Each subsequent reading has, I think, made me a better physician.

★   ★   ★

I hope that these brief reviews lead you to read these five beautifully written books. All define and expand the dimensions of courage.

WORKS CITED

Bauby, Jean-Dominique. *The Diving Bell and the Butterfly*. New York: Knopf; 1998.

Carver, Raymond. *A New Path to the Waterfall*. New York: Atlantic Monthly Press; 1989.

Daudet, Alphonse. *In the Land of Pain*. Julian Barnes, ed. and trans. New York: Knopf; 2002.

Lomax, Eric. *The Railway Man*. New York: W.W. Norton; 1995.

Price, Reynolds. *A Whole New Life: An Illness and a Healing*. New York: Atheneum; 1994.